# EMERGENCY DISPATCHING

## A Medical Communicator's Guide

Susi B. Steele

*MedStar Ambulance / Texas Lifeline Corporation*
*Fort Worth, Texas*

**REGENTS/PRENTICE HALL**
Englewood Cliffs, New Jersey 07632

**Library of Congress Cataloging-in-Publication Data**

Steele, Susi B.
   Emergency dispatching : a medical communicator's guide / Susi B. Steele.
      p.    cm.
   Includes index.
   ISBN 0-89303-835-0
   1. Ambulance service -- Dispatching.  2. Communication in emergency medicine.  I. Title
   [DNLM: 1. Emergency Medical Service Communication Systems -- organization & administration.  2. Emergency Medical Technicians. WX 215 S814e]
RA995.S74   1993
362.1'88 -- dc20
DNLM/DLC
for Library of Congress                                       93-49634
                                                                                 CIP

Editorial/production supervision,
  interior design, and electronic production: *Julie Boddorf*
Cover design: *Marianne Frasco*
Cover photo: *Robert D. Steele*
Prepress buyer: *Ilene Levy*
Manufacturing buyer: *Ed O'Dougherty*
Acquisitions editor: *Natalie Anderson*
Editorial assistant: *Louise Fullam*

***Notice:*** *The author and the publisher of this book have taken care to make certain that the procedures are correct and compatible with standards generally acceptable at the time of publication. Nevertheless, as new information becomes available, changes in procedures become necessary. The readers are advised to consult with their medical advisors in accordance with local laws and regulations. The publisher and author disclaim any liability, loss, injury, or damage incurred as a consequence, directly or indirectly, of the use and application of any of the contents of this book.*

© 1993 by REGENTS/PRENTICE HALL
A Division of Simon & Schuster
Englewood Cliffs, New Jersey 07632

All rights reserved. No part of this book may be
reproduced, in any form or by any means,
without permission in writing from the publisher.

Printed in the United States of America

10  9  8  7  6  5  4  3  2  1

ISBN   0-89303-835-0

PRENTICE-HALL INTERNATIONAL (UK) LIMITED, London
PRENTICE-HALL OF AUSTRALIA PTY. LIMITED, Sydney
PRENTICE-HALL CANADA INC., Toronto
PRENTICE-HALL HISPANOAMERICANA, S.A., Mexico
PRENTICE-HALL OF INDIA PRIVATE LIMITED, New Delhi
PRENTICE-HALL OF JAPAN, INC., Tokyo
SIMON & SCHUSTER ASIA PTE. LTD., Singapore
EDITORA PRENTICE-HALL DO BRASIL, LTDA., Rio de Janeiro

*This book is respectfully dedicated
to the Best of the Best*

*The MedStar Medical Communications Team*

| | |
|---|---|
| *Peter Attwell* | *Leslie Gilliland* |
| *Keith Armstrong* | *Joe Goodall* |
| *Ed Bodiford* | *Jimmy Hudgins* |
| *Anna Brown* | *Kay Hurdle* |
| *Valerie Carson* | *Starrett Keele* |
| *Lori Damron* | *Joe Martin* |
| *Mark Dana* | *David Mowrey* |
| *Marsha Felsinger* | *Charlene Robertson* |

*and always to*

*MyBob*

# CONTENTS

INTRODUCTION     xv

THE MEDICAL COMMUNICATOR'S CREED     xvii

**1 THE ROLE OF THE MEDICAL COMMUNICATOR IN TODAY'S EMS SYSTEM**     1

An Historical Perspective   1

Old-Style Management Structures   1

The Organization of Progressive EMS Systems   3
*The Importance of Medical Control,* 5
*Other Important Elements in System Design:
The Roles of Ancillary Personnel,* 5

Industry Trends: Reintroducing the Human Element   6
*In the Beginning,* 6
*The Growth of the EMS System,* 6
*The Emergence of National Performance Standards,* 7

A Change in Perspective: Understanding the Big Picture   8

Commonly Used Terms   8

Making Educated Choices: Maintaining a Balance   9

The Importance of Aggressive Quality Assurance Planning  9

The Changing Role of the Medical Communicator  9
*Take Dispatchers and Dinosaurs . . ., 10
Add Some Telphone Triage . . ., 10
Throw in Some System Status Management . . ., 11
And It Comes Out Here!, 12*

Our New Public Image  12

Special Concentration Needs in the Communications Center  13

Summary and Review  15

## 2 ATTITUDES AND MOTIVATION  17

Establishing Your Priorities  17
*First, Last, and Always: Patient Care
and Customer Satisfaction, 17
Providing for Field Care-Givers, 18*

Confidentiality and Integrity  18

Maintaining a Positive Attitude  19

Summary and Review  24

## 3 THE OPERATION OF THE COMMUNICATIONS CENTER  25

Setting Yourself Up to Win  25

The Location of the Communications Center  27

Designing the Physical Layout  27

Setting Departmental Standards  28

Protecting Your Position  30

Types of Personalities in the Communications Center  30

Scheduling and Staffing  35
*Structuring the Hours, 36
Alternates versus Full-Time Communicators, 39*

Rotating Through the Positions  39

Cooperation  40

Practical Problem Solving: Where's Your Sense of Humor?  40

Shift Assignments and Advancement Within the Department  42

Making Critical Decisions  42

Summary and Review  42

# Contents

**4 SYSTEM STATUS MANAGEMENT**    44

   What Is It, Anyway?   44

   Goals of System Status Management   45

   Off to a Rocky Start: What Happened Here?   45

   Learning from the Experience of Others:
   Although We Are Special, We're Not That Different   46

   Choosing Smart Over Stupid   47

   Making Intelligent Decisions   48

   Definitions of Common Terms   49

   Using the Results of Call Demand Analyses   51

   Lost and Added Unit Hours   51

   Response Time Reporting   54

   Tracking the Wild Exception   57

   Unit Deployment and Post Selection   57
      *The Strategy of Ambulance Placement, 57*
      *Making Your Post Selections, 59*
      *Consideration of System Levels, 61*
      *Writing the Plan, 61*
      *Implementing the New Deployment Plan, 61*

   Measuring Productivity   63

   Summary and Review   64

**5 ROLES AND RESPONSIBILITIES OF THE MEDICAL COMMUNICATOR**    65

   Initial Contact with the Public   65

   Channeling Communications   66

   Concern for Crew Safety   66

   Policies and Procedures   66

   System Status Planning and On-Line Management   66

   Geographic Knowledge   67

   Knowledge of Your Equipment   67

   Handling Routine Radio and Telephone Traffic   68

   Receiving and Processing Call Information   68

   Telephone Triage and Remote-Directed Intervention   68

Resource Management 68

Range of Services 69

Interfacing with Other Departments and Agencies 69

System Status and System Compliance with Obligations 69

Quality Assurance 69

Working as a Team Player 70

Instant Replay 70

Activities Inappropriate to the Medical Communicator 71

Summary and Review 72

## 6 BASIC COMMUNICATION AND TELECOMMUNICATION THEORY 73

The Four Components of Communication 73

Training versus Natural Talent 73

If I Can Speak English, How Hard Can This Be? 74

Behavior Modification Technique 75
*Poor Listening Habits, 75*
*Positive Listening Habits 75*
*Improved Speaking Habits, 76*

The Challenge of a New Perspective 77

Communication versus Telecommunication 77

Working with a Handicap 78

The Spoken Word versus Gesture 79

The Nature of the Medical Communicator 80

Summary and Review 80

## 7 BASIC TELEPHONE TECHNIQUES 81

The Telephone as a Tool 81

The Five Things You Should Never Say to a Customer 81

Basic Telephone Techniques 83

The Speed of the Response: First Impressions Count 83

Communications Center Overload 84

Answering the Emergency Telephone Line 85

Answering the Non-emergency Telephone Line   86

Handling Complaints   87

A Note About Evaluations   88

Don't Hang Up!   88

Summary and Review   89

## 8 TELEPHONE TRIAGE AND REMOTE INTERVENTION   90

What Is Telephone Triage?   90

Priority Dispatching Defined   90

What Is Remote Intervention?   90

The Philosophy Behind the Change   91

Common Objections and Misconceptions   91

Call Prioritization versus Call Screening   92

Practical Guidelines for Establishing Algorithms   92

Summary and Review   94

## 9 ADVANCED TELECOMMUNICATIONS TECHNIQUES   95

First, Learn the Basics   95

Common Terms and Principles   95
*Total Acknowledgment, 95*
*The "Half-Ack", 97*
*The Comment, 97*
*The Origination, 97*
*The Hysteria Threshold, 98*
*Repetitive Persistence, 98*
*"Freak" and "Refreak", 99*

Attitude Adjustment   100

Summary and Review   100

## 10 THE PSYCHOLOGY OF DEALING WITH THE PERSON IN CRISIS   101

Components of the Hysterical Response   101

Attack and Counterattack   102

Categorizing Our Callers   103

Building a Mental Picture   103

Someone Else's Shoes   104

Dealing with the Elderly Caller   105

How to Talk to Children   106

How Important is Your Reaction to Panic?   107

Summary and Review   107

## 11 RECEIVING AND PROCESSING THE CALL FOR ASSISTANCE   108

Review: First Contact with the Public   108

Provision of Medical Information   108

Timely and Appropriate Assignment of Resources   109

Coordination with Other Public Safety Services   109

Eliciting and Recording Dispatch Information: Answering the Telephone   109

The Three Essential Elements   109

Receiving the Nonemergency Call   110

Key Questions   111

Third-Party Limitations   112

Continuing the Process   113

Offering a Different Kind of Help   113

Following Through   114

Summary and Review   114

## 12 RADIO COMMUNICATIONS   115

Who Are You and Why Are You Here?   115

Another Change in Perspective   116

Radio Codes and Signals or Plain English?   116

Radio Operations: A Procedural Overview   117

Pre-Alerting Appropriate Field Units   118

Dispatching the Response   119

Acknowledging Unit Transmissions   120

Making Post Move-Ups   120

Summary and Review   121

## 13 MEDICOLEGAL ISSUES IN EMERGENCY MEDICAL DISPATCHING — 122

Overview: Welcome to the Real World  122

Common Mistakes: Danger Zones for Litigation  123

Important Legal Terms and Concepts as They Apply to Medical Dispatchers  124
- *Duty, 124*
- *Negligence, 124*
- *The Prudent Action Rule, 125*
- *The Emergency Rule, 125*
- *Foreseeability, 126*
- *Deviation from Protocols, 126*
- *Special Relationships, 127*
- *Detrimental Reliance, 127*

Future Shock  127

Summary and Review  128

## 14 DOCUMENTATION AND REPORTING TECHNIQUES — 129

A Change in Focus  129

The Increased Need for Documentation  129

Practical Techniques and Applications  130

Audio Recordings as Documentation  130

Time Stamping Status Changes and Important Events  130

Types of Reporting and Documentation: Different Needs, Different Methods  131
- *Medical Information: Documentation of the Response, 132*
- *Legal Documentation, 135*
- *Maintaining Community Health, 142*
- *Recording Data for Administrative Purposes, 145*

The Commitment to Excellence, 146

Summary and Review  147

## 15 PUBLIC RELATIONS — 148

What Is It? (What Are They?): A Question of Semantics  148

Dealing with the Media: The Nature of the Process  149
- *Back to Basic Communication, 149*
- *Changing Your Attitude Toward Media Representatives, 149*
- *Practical Guidelines for Release of Information, 151*
- *Major Media Events, 151*

Public Education  152

*The Lack of Citizen Planning, 152*
*Common Barriers to Change, 154*
*Why Bother?, 155*
*Educating the Public: When to Try, 155*
*What to Do and How to Do It, 156*

Contributing to Customer Satisfaction 158

Summary and Review 160

## 16 QUALITY ASSURANCE AND QUALITY IMPROVEMENT IN EMERGENCY MEDICAL DISPATCHING 161

The Need for Quality Assurance 161

Utilizing the Team Approach 161

Quality Assurance in Emergency Medical Service 162

Types of Errors in the Communications Center 162

Medical Control 163

Standardization of Telephone Procedures 164

Position Statements and Procedures 164

Candidate Selection 165

Setting Minimum Prerequisite Standards 165

The Selection Process 166

Candidate Testing 174

The Initial Training Process 176

Interim Performance Appraisals 186

Written Medical Communicator Examinations: Establishing a System to Evaluate Technical Knowledge 186
*Levels of Testing, 188*

Other Types of Testing 190
*Psychological Testing, 190*
*Intelligence Testing, 190*

Attitude Surveys 190

Analyzing and Interpreting Test Results: Establishing the Proper Perspective 191
*Measures of Relationship: Common Terms, 191*
*Measures of Variability, 193*
*Standard Deviation from Mean, 193*

Training, Retraining and Continuing Education 193
*Initial Training, 194*

*Remedial Retraining, 194*
*Continuing Education, 195*

Audio Tape Reviews 197

Routine Performance Evaluations 200

Summary and Review 200

## 17 STRESS MANAGEMENT FOR THE MEDICAL COMMUNICATOR 202

Components of the Stress Reaction 202

What Is Stress? 203

Reinforcing Our Public Image 203

Common Stress Factors for Medical Communicators 204

Signs and Symptoms of Stress Overload and Burnout 208

Words to Live By 213

Managing Stress Overload to Avoid Burnout 214
*Positive Stress Management Techniques, 215*

Allowing for Change 216

Professional Assistance 217

Critical Incident Stress Management 218

Summary and Review 220

## 18 DISASTER PLANNING 221

How to Avoid Hosting Your Own Disaster 221

Why We Plan Before the Fact 221

The Unique Needs of Medical Communicators 222

The Hazards of Working in the Spotlight 223

Planning for the Communications Center 223

The Ten Critical Steps 224

Setting Practical Goals for the Communications Center 237

The Ultimate Goals 238

Summary and Review 238

GLOSSARY OF TERMS 240

INDEX 247

# INTRODUCTION

There has always been a certain mystique surrounding the extraordinarily competent dispatcher ("We don't know exactly what she does, and we're not sure exactly how she does it, but damn, she's good!"). For years, the really *good* dispatchers have jealously guarded the secrets of their success. They have taught newcomers in the technical requirements of the job, and left out training in the areas of communications and "people" skills which made them exceptional. As trainers and administrators, we have expected our communicators to somehow magically acquire the knowledge they need to do the job; however, we have never *taught* them. When I began looking for research material to provide to the medical dispatchers in my system, I found that, for the most part, what I wanted simply didn't exist in written form. I believe that we need to start sharing our ideas, in order to once again improve the quality of patient care provided nationwide.

This text is the result of my attempt to give my system's medical communicators the education, support, and protection they deserve. It was developed to help them feel secure, and to keep them safe. It is intended to be used as a teaching tool, and a "jumping-off" place for new ideas.

The focus of the text may be confusing to some; first, it seems to be speaking to line dispatchers, then to line supervisors, then to system managers, and then to line communicators again. This continual change in perspective is deliberate; in most systems, line communicators act in a supervisory capacity each shift they work, and need to become much more involved in decision making and quality improvement. I believe it is also time for line communicators to take some ownership in their own field of expertise, and to contribute to the development and refinement of their own job descriptions.

As for the informal (sometimes very casual, sometimes silly, and occasionally downright disrespectful) style in which this text is written, consider this: If you are employed or seek employment as a medical communicator, you occupy a critically important position in the emergency medical service industry. *Emergency medical service exists, by definition, in a constant, continuing state of crisis.* When you choose a profession that encounters more than its share of the ridiculous, you had best find some functional way to rationalize the absurdity; otherwise, it will eat you alive. To survive in this industry, you have to develop a sense of humor. Besides, this is the way I really talk. If you don't like it, write your own book. Go ahead. *I dare you.*

## ACKNOWLEDGMENTS

The author gratefully acknowledges the help and support of the following professionals who, sometimes unaware, taught by their examples:

Tom Morgan, Glen Roberts, and Kurt Williams
*Hartson Medical Service, San Diego, California*

Bob Forbuss and Janet Smith
*Mercy Ambulance Service, Las Vegas, Nevada*

Jack Stout
*The Fourth Party, Inc., Fairfax, Virginia*

Jeff Clawson, MD
*Medical Priority Consultants, Inc., Salt Lake City, Utah*

And my friends

Steve Athey
*MedStar/Texas Lifeline Corporation, Fort Worth, Texas*
Who made me start and finish this project,

And Deb Silkwood
*Hartson Medical Service, San Diego, California*
Who kept me sane in between.

Thanks, y'all

## The Medical Communicator's Creed

*We, the professionals of emergency medical communications,
are dedicated to providing the highest quality care, whatever the need.*

*We are, first and foremost, medical professionals. We are an
integral part of the worldwide network that provides care and comfort
to the sick and injured. We are committed to continually
improving the standards of pre-hospital care.*

*We are people of honesty and integrity. We will respect the dignity
and preserve the privacy of all those into whose lives we enter, never
revealing what we witness in those lives unless required by law.*

*We are people helping people. We will serve continuously
and unselfishly, sharing our medical knowledge with any who
may benefit from what we have learned. We will accept from
ourselves and each other nothing less than excellence. Our reward
will be the knowledge that we have taken every opportunity
to positively impact each life into which we enter, making
this world a better place for all.*

# Chapter 1

# THE ROLE OF THE MEDICAL COMMUNICATOR IN TODAY'S EMS SYSTEM

*"Genius ain't anything more than elegant common sense."*
— *Josh Billings*

## AN HISTORICAL PERSPECTIVE

In the "good old days" of emergency medical care and transportation services, we made our own rules, and we made them up as we went along. We were such foreign animals that it did not occur to anyone, including us, that we should function by the basic principles used to successfully manage other types of companies in other industry categories. The organizational structure of any EMS service was very simple and straightforward. The "big boss" was at the top of the pile; everybody else was underneath. No one told the big boss, whether he (and it was always a he) was a fire chief or the president of a private enterprise, what to do or how to do it. This typical structure was a natural development, which grew from the fact that no one knew who we were, what we did, or how we did it. As we gained prominence and recognition with the public and our expertise and liabilities increased, our system structures became more complex, although not necessarily better.

## OLD-STYLE MANAGEMENT STRUCTURES

The form of a typical "old-style" EMS system (see Figure 1.1) included these elements:

- The *big boss*: the chief of the department, the president of the company, the owner, the chief executive officer, the director, etc.

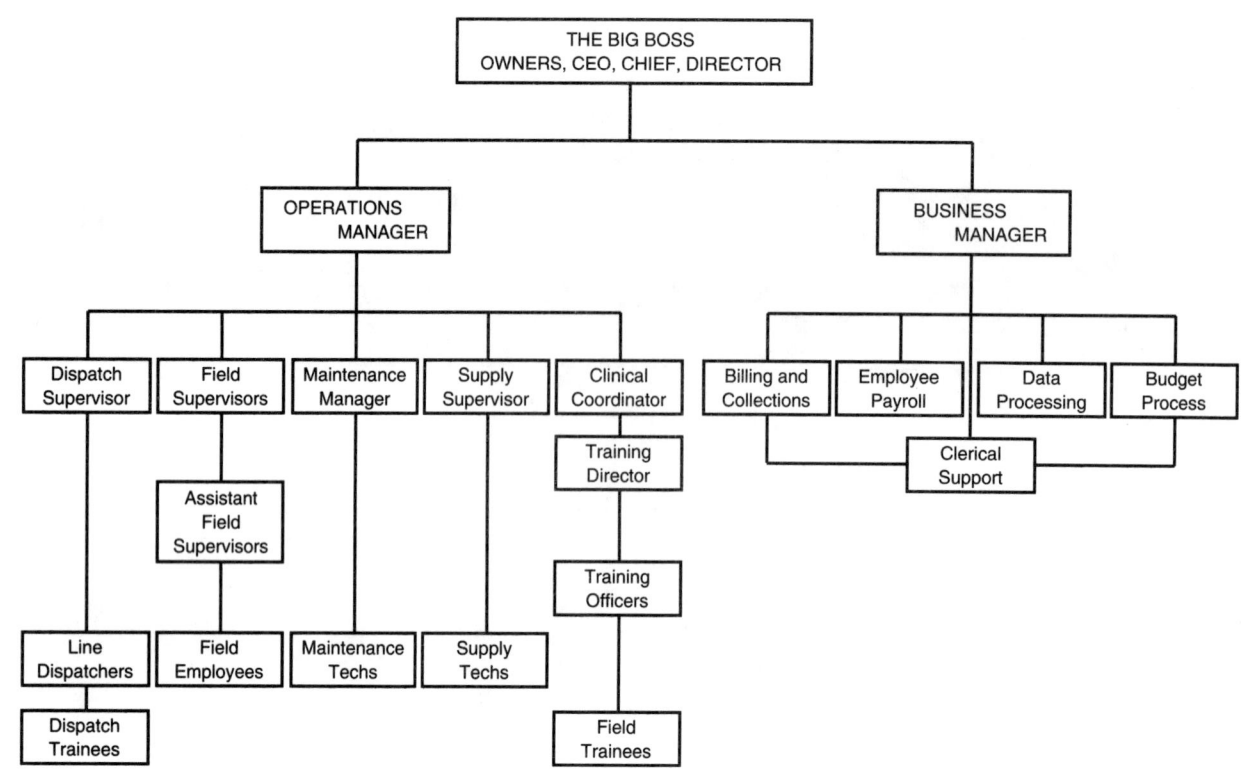

Figure 1.1  Typical "old-style" EMS management structure

The big boss sat in a big office making big plans and doing big things, although nobody knew exactly what those big things were. He came out occasionally to hand down a new directive which made sense to almost no one. The big boss made all the critical policy decisions alone, although his knowledge of the state of his own system depended completely on input from the operations and financial managers. The big boss was either a genius or an idiot, depending upon how much accessibility he allowed by the field and line personnel (familiarity breeds contempt).

- The *financial director*: the business manager, comptroller, etc. The financial director, poor thing, usually had no medical training other than coding Medicare claims. The financial director was universally looked down on by those actually providing patient care. Her/his expertise was in the area of accounting or business, and therefore she or he couldn't possibly be as important as those involved in operations. The business section of the service crunched numbers and completed the paperwork that the people on the field side of the operation were too busy and too specifically skilled to do. The financial director was responsible for budgeting (which never gave us all that we wanted), collections (which were never high enough), payroll (our paychecks were always wrong), marketing (which we were sure we could have handled better), data processing (where an incredible number of errors were made), and so on. The "business" aspect of any organization was kept carefully separate from the operations side.

- The *operations manager* was responsible for everything the financial department was not. She/he was, directly or indirectly, charged with supervision of both field personnel and dispatchers, hiring and firing of personnel, training and continuing education, maintenance and supply. The operations manager designed and implemented shift schedules, and controlled staffing levels. Operations managers literally managed every aspect of the system's operations, and answered only to the big boss.

## THE ORGANIZATION OF PROGRESSIVE EMS SYSTEMS

*"No one can walk backward into the future."*
— Joseph Hergesheimer

As our profession became more visible and better grounded, the demands placed upon us by our customers, the public, changed and increased. With more visibility came more potential for litigation. With more understanding of our profession and more respect for the service we provide came stricter demands for high-quality medical care. As our place in the medical community changed, our organizational needs changed. Our methods of structuring have become both more realistic and more practical as our experience base has grown. Today's EMS system welcomes guidance and informational input from a variety of sources (Figure 1.2). The elements necessary to function as a highly productive, highly efficient system include:

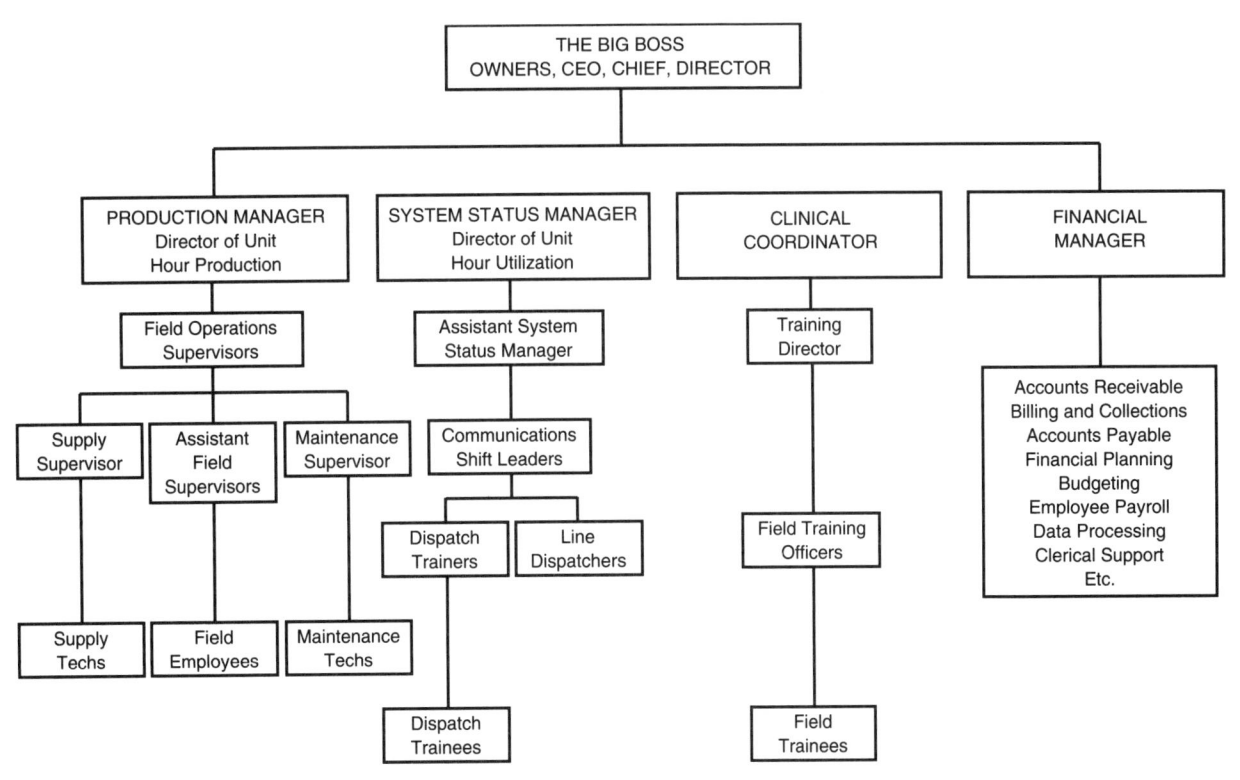

Figure 1.2  *New EMS management structure*

- The *big boss*. There will always be a need for that one person or group that functions as a single entity (i.e., board of directors), to accept the final responsibility for everything that happens in an EMS system. The big boss directs the managers (or deputy chiefs, department heads, supervisors, etc.). However, the big boss is more secure now, and recognizes the ultimate profitability and protection gained from accepting input and guidance from experts in other fields: legal, medical, financial, business.
- The *system status manager* (SSM) is a relatively new addition to the structure. She/he is responsible for maintaining the healthy status of the system, and identifies, defines, and directs unit hour utilization. The SSM analyzes historical data and predicts future call volume, geographic demand, and staffing needs. Clearly defined unit hour requirements are passed to the production manager, who builds schedules to satisfy those needs. The SSM is responsible for data management and reporting. She/he reports directly to the big boss.
- The *communications supervisor* is responsible for the attitude, motivation, standard of performance, and direction of communications as a department. She/he completes the initial information-gathering process and provides on-site supervision and support to the medical dispatchers. She/he is an advocate for the communicators. The communications supervisor reports directly to the system status manager.
- The *production manager* now serves as the director of unit hour production. She/he takes the demands identified by the system status manager and forms them into practical, workable procedures. She/he is ultimately responsible for all field personnel, maintenance, and supply. The production manager reports directly to the big boss.
- *Field operations supervisors* manage the day-to-day needs of the field care-givers. They help to interpret, implement, and enforce policies and procedures for field personnel, and provide ongoing evaluations of their employees' job performance. They are called field supervisors because they belong in the field, not in an office somewhere crunching numbers. Field supervisors report directly to the production manager.
- The *financial director* is still responsible for patient billing, collection of accounts, budgeting, data processing, payroll, and general data management and record-keeping. She/he is now encouraged to fill a more active role in directing the activities of the provider, thus contributing to the maintenance of a healthy financial status of the system.
- The *fleet maintenance manager* is responsible for the general upkeep of the units, maintaining records to satisfy warranty requirements, and devising a schedule for effective preventative maintenance on the vehicles. She/he may also design training programs for field personnel to assist them in caring for the ambulances.

- The *supply supervisor* handles inventory control, product testing and evaluation, and ordering of both hard equipment and disposable supplies. She/he also streamlines and improves resupply procedures to decrease the amount of resupply downtime in the system.

### The Importance of Medical Control

In these days of high standards for medical care providers, *medical control* is an essential part of any responsible EMS system. Medical control is accomplished through the activities of four entities: the clinical coordinator, the medical director, the physicians' advisory group, and the training director.

The *clinical coordinator* is employed by the system to monitor and improve clinical performance. She/he reviews medical care given, and acts as medical liaison between field care-givers and the other elements of the professional medical community. The clinical coordinator supervises the activities of the training director and the field training officers. This position reports directly to the big boss, and indirectly to the medical community as a whole.

The *medical director* is a physician employed by the system to provide overall medical direction and to liaise with other physicians and medical personnel outside the system. Field care-givers give scheduled drugs and utilize standing orders under the license of the physician medical director.

The *physicians' advisory group* is made up of area physicians, ideally those specializing in emergency medicine. This group reviews standing orders, prioritization and pre-arrival protocols, and the like, compares these with local, state, and national standards, and helps to formulate policies that affect medical care. The participants also review selected cases and make suggestions for improvement.

The *training director* may be either the same person as the clinical coordinator, or may report directly to that position. The training director administers initial training of field personnel and maintains records of certification levels and expiration dates. She/he is responsible for training the system's first responders and for structuring a comprehensive and workable continuing education program.

### Other Important Elements in System Design: The Roles of Ancillary Personnel

In addition to the positions just described that directly impact field and dispatch personnel, there are others that, though they may impact the employees indirectly, are no less important.

- The *public relations* or public information director works with

various media representatives to maintain a healthy public image for the system.
- The *benefits administrator* designs employee benefits packages and assists employees' utilization of those benefits.
- *Employee support groups and action teams* perform every function from reviewing motor vehicle accidents involving ambulances to providing immediate emotional support for the employee in crisis. Employee-directed programs are strongly recommended to increase employees' involvement and ownership in the system, to improve morale, and to find practical, workable solutions to problems.
- Various *consultants* in the areas of the law, finance, and system design contribute to the general health of the system, and help to find innovative solutions for real or impending problems. Doing something a certain way as the result of soliciting an expert opinion is immeasurably preferable to continuing a process or procedure because "It's always been done that way."

## INDUSTRY TRENDS: REINTRODUCING THE HUMAN ELEMENT

*"They be blind leaders of the blind. And if the blind lead the blind, both shall fall into the ditch."*
— New Testament, Matt. 15:14

### In the Beginning

Emergency medical service (EMS) in most parts of the country had its origins in ambulance transportation provided by funeral homes. In the early days of ambulance service, patient care was minimal, calltaking and dispatching were often part-time functions performed by clerical personnel, and "customer service" was almost completely unheard of. Eventually, advanced life support units staffed by paramedics qualified to provide definitive patient care were introduced; it was at this point that true "emergency" medical service in most service areas began.

### The Growth of the EMS System

Although advanced life support (ALS) units were on the streets in many areas more than 20 years ago, a true *system* of emergency medical response did not begin to emerge in most areas until several years later. Prior to that time, a field paramedic's ability to give definitive care to her/his patient often depended on the individual paramedic's professional relationship with the physician answering the EMS radio at the facility of choice. Paramedics were hired, retained, and made advancements within EMS services based on extremely subjective criteria. In-house (agency or department administered) programs to monitor adherence to performance criteria were almost nonexistent. Training, certification, and levels of competence required were usually no more demanding or structured than was dictated by any state's health department standards. Similarly, performance standards in the dispatch center were largely unidentified, and compliance with those requirements that were identified remained unenforced. The first question asked of a person who called for help was, *"Is this an emergency?"* The decision to dispatch the call or shunt it to a nonemergency service was made solely on the caller's answer to that one question. No further prioritization was attempted, and no pre-arrival instructions were given. Response times were averaged, and documentation was sketchy, at best. Subsidies in cities served by private sector EMS systems were high, and collection rates for services rendered were low; the financial states of private EMS services were almost universally precarious. It was a widely accepted belief that no entity which provided emergency medical service would ever operate at a profit.

### The Emergence of National Performance Standards

As the function of emergency medical care-givers began to mature as a profession, paramedicine began to attract the attention of those professionals highly skilled in business, financial, and administrative techniques, as well as those intensively trained in emergency medicine. At about the same time that real, functional EMS systems began to emerge nationwide, the principles of system status management, performance-based service contracts, and overall high levels of system efficiency began to be accepted as the national standard for EMS services. At the same time, more advanced, more complicated patient management techniques became available to field care-givers, and medical prioritization gained national prominence in dispatch centers across the country. More and more, emphasis was moved away from subjective standards based on personalities and open to interpretation, and toward strict adherence to regulations structured to ensure adequate technical performance in every possible situation.

The results of this shift in focus to technical excellence were dramatic. With the new emphasis on system efficiency, in many areas the human element lost definite ground, although field care of the high-risk patient improved. Great importance was placed on saving the life of the super-critical patient; the issues of simple patient discomfort and patient or facility inconvenience were pushed aside while we handled the "real emergencies." Similarly, compliance with contractual and medically necessary response time requirements was stressed, and, in many parts of the country, system status management was implemented and administered very strictly by rules formulated for nonspecific, often hypothetical service areas. The responsibilities of medical dispatchers were increased; again, the acceptability of the medical communicators' performance was gauged by their adherence to guidelines that originated in a distant or hypothetical service market. Little or no customization was performed to allow for demographic differences in service areas. Results and performance levels that could be measured and documented on paper were pursued with a vengeance. The pendulum that started with "gut instinct" patient care and "make it up as you go" dispatching procedures had completed its swing to the other extreme.

## A CHANGE IN PERSPECTIVE: UNDERSTANDING THE BIG PICTURE

Now that we have achieved technical excellence, established responsible guidelines for performance capabilities for the various positions in EMS, and instituted a reasonable, maintainable system of checks and balances to constantly analyze and improve our overall performance as EMS providers, we must take the next logical developmental step. We must combine the best of both extremes previously outlined, and reach and maintain a balanced perspective of the services we provide.

## COMMONLY USED TERMS

At this point, we must examine three key phrases frequently used in our profession: *patient care, customer service, and customer satisfaction* (Figure 1.3). These terms are usually very poorly defined, even in the minds of those who work in the industry.

It is obvious that *patient care* is the sum of the hands-on medical care provided by your system's field employees. However, it is now widely recognized that the medical communicator also provides patient care. Although you may not be able to *see* your patient, you can still dramatically impact the outcome of any specific incident for that patient. You can effectively, with telephone triage and pre-arrival instructions, change the practical response time from four or six or eight minutes to zero. *Patient care begins the minute that conversation begins with the caller.*

*Customer service* includes all the little things that your system does to accommodate the human needs of your customers and clients. Customer service can, and does, include everything from the establishment of a dress or uniform code for field employees to the implementation of easily understood billing practices. In this area, everything that your system does matters.

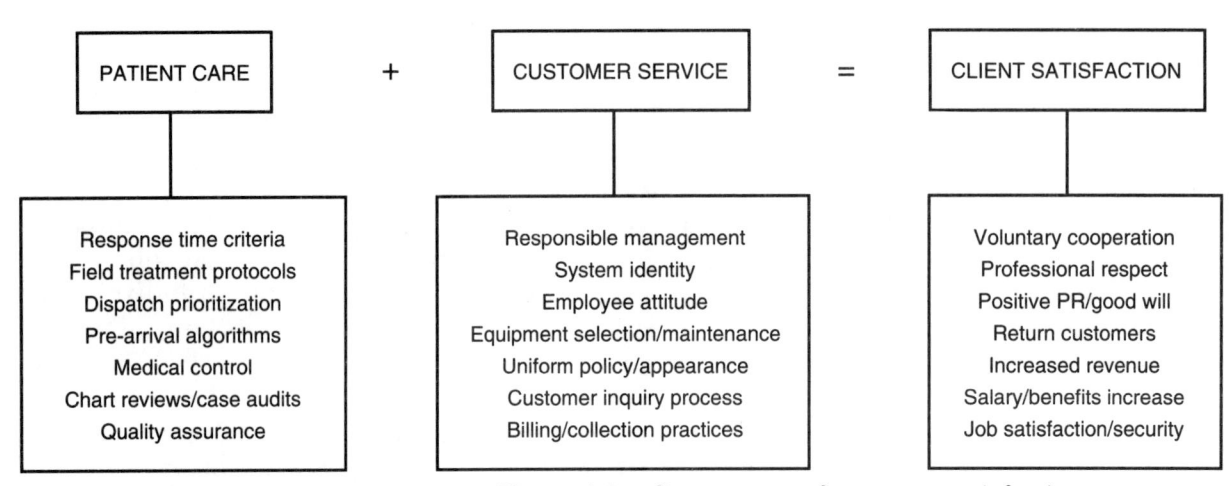

| PATIENT CARE | + | CUSTOMER SERVICE | = | CLIENT SATISFACTION |
|---|---|---|---|---|
| Response time criteria<br>Field treatment protocols<br>Dispatch prioritization<br>Pre-arrival algorithms<br>Medical control<br>Chart reviews/case audits<br>Quality assurance | | Responsible management<br>System identity<br>Employee attitude<br>Equipment selection/maintenance<br>Uniform policy/appearance<br>Customer inquiry process<br>Billing/collection practices | | Voluntary cooperation<br>Professional respect<br>Positive PR/good will<br>Return customers<br>Increased revenue<br>Salary/benefits increase<br>Job satisfaction/security |

Figure 1.3 *Components of customer satisfaction*

*Customer satisfaction* is the end product of all your efforts in the areas of patient care and customer service. Customer satisfaction must be strived for and maintained to provide any degree of job security for the system's personnel. If your system consistently provides both high-quality patient care and courteous, disciplined customer service, customer satisfaction will be the inevitable result.

## MAKING EDUCATED CHOICES: MAINTAINING A BALANCE

When we place undue emphasis on caring for critical emergency patients at the expense of all others, we lose our ability to provide widespread customer satisfaction with our system. *We become out of balance.* When we place excessive importance on response time compliance to the exclusion of all else, and utilize statistics alone to build our system status plan, we increase the number of post move-ups made, thereby increasing the work load on our field crews and correspondingly, increasing their fatigue levels. *Again, we become out of balance.*

Your goal now, as an individual, as a department, as an organization, and as an industry, should be to reintroduce the human element into your system, combining it with your proven technical excellence to provide to your customers a network of services that is complete, customized, and addresses each and every client need.

## THE IMPORTANCE OF AGGRESSIVE QUALITY ASSURANCE PLANNING

A comprehensive, competitive *quality assurance* (QA) or *quality improvement* program is absolutely necessary in the operation of every present-day EMS system. While detailed suggestions for structuring quality assurance plans specifically for communications departments are discussed at length in Chapter 19 of this text, these basic points should be noted:

*First*, that employee involvement is the most critical element impacting the success or failure of any QA program.
*Second*, that if every case or every chart is not reviewed, eventually a decrease in an employee's competency level will be missed by managers and will result in endangerment, complaint, or litigation.
*Third*, that in today's business and professional climate, we must not only be able to perform our roles in emergency medical service to meet or exceed a high performance standard, *we must be able to prove on demand that we can do so.*

## THE CHANGING ROLE OF THE MEDICAL COMMUNICATOR

*"Dear, dear! How queer everything is to-day! And yesterday things went on just as usual. I wonder if I've been changed in the night? But if I'm not the same, then the next question is, Who in the world am I?"*
— *Alice, from "Alice's Adventures in Wonderland" by Lewis Carroll*

### Take Dispatchers and Dinosaurs...

Generally, when a new word is coined or a new phrase is created, it is given a specific meaning. As time passes and the new word is used, it accumulates some of the "baggage" of language. It acquires secondary or hidden meanings, and begins to carry with it mental associations, either positive or negative, that may be completely unrelated to its definition in the dictionary. Words create a mental picture in the mind of the listener; that image reflects not just the actual meaning of the word, but also any implied associations.

*Dispatcher,* although not an archaic word, is not new to our vocabulary. "To dispatch" means "to issue or send forth." Initially, an inferred association suggested that the sending would be accomplished with speed. These are all positive connotations; however, they completely miss the mark in attempting to describe the many functions that we perform in EMS today. Dispatchers are used in many industries. There is a dispatcher who sends the taxi to pick you up at the airport. A dispatcher keeps track of the drivers for a delivery system. Dispatchers send the exterminator to your house when you schedule an appointment, and, when one of our computer keyboards malfunctions, dispatchers notify the technicians with our support service. In the early days of EMS, when ambulance services advertised themselves to be "radio dispatched, oxygen equipped," dispatchers dispatched ambulances, too. The current "feeling" attached to the word is usually neutral, since very few people have any idea at all what we do and how we do it.

In those beginning years of our industry, a dispatcher, by the simplest definition of the job title, could adequately perform the job to which she/he was assigned. Response times were averaged, and virtually no responsibility for extended response times was placed with the dispatcher. Little or no telephone interrogation took place; when questioning *was* performed, the frequent result was *call screening* rather than *call prioritization*. The concept of pre-arrival instructions did not exist. Field units had assigned districts, and did not move outside their boundaries except to transport patients. In many systems, no medical training was required to dispatch ambulances. In some systems, the dispatch office was routinely used as a "dumping ground" for field employees who, due to illness or injury, had been placed on light duty. In others, dispatch was considered simply an extended clerical function (unfortunately, in many small communities where fire, police, and EMS dispatch are combined, this attitude still exists).

### Add Some Telephone Triage...

When the concepts of *medical interrogation* and *call prioritization* were introduced by Dr. Jeff Clawson in Salt Lake City, Utah, the entire scope of the dispatcher's duties began to change. As Clawson's techniques proved effective in positively impacting the final outcome for patients in the Salt Lake system, more and more systems nationwide began to adopt his training and performance criteria in their own communications centers. In some areas, the local algorithms for medical dispatch were originally written for nonmedical personnel, and were performed by lay persons. In some systems, it is now believed that medically trained communicators with field experience have two immediate advantages: first, they aren't operating "blind" through the process of attempting to determine what is wrong with the patient; and second, their field experience gives them an edge in identifying the particulars of the patient's condition, identifying scene access and hazards, and anticipating the needs of the responding field crews.

Throw in Some System Status Management . . .

The use of system status management began to grow in popularity at about the same time that innovative systems were beginning to experiment with call prioritization and pre-arrival instructions. This added another component to what started as a simple, uncomplicated list of job duties. Now the communicator was required to know, at any time and on demand, exactly where each and every unit in the system was, what task that unit was performing, and what the estimated time was until the completion of that task. She/he became directly involved in the chain of responsibility for extended response times. As the duties and responsibilities of the communicator increased and broadened in scope, the image associated with the position changed.

The well-rounded, performance-motivated medical communicator functions by default at a supervisory level, *even if that supervisory status is not specifically defined in the communicator's job description.* The respect that goes with a supervisory-level position will not be given to you simply because you demand it. You must earn it by holding yourself accountable for your actions, your attitude, and your demeanor. You must hold yourself to a rigid performance standard, and allow yourself to be governed by a thoroughly professional attitude every shift that you work.

In any system, at the point when the medical communicator begins to function in a supervisory capacity, a radical emotional separation between field and communications personnel begins to occur. The role of the communicator abruptly changes. Previously, the communicator was seen as a nonauthoritative personality who simply provided information to the field crews when a response was to be made. Now, the communicator becomes an authority figure. With the implementation of medical prioritization, the dispatcher becomes a *medical communicator* who tells crews in what mode they will make their responses. With the implementation of system status management, the dispatcher becomes a *system status controller.* The system status controller follows a proscribed deployment plan by giving nonnegotiable instructions to field personnel who, without forethought and planning, frequently do not understand the reasons behind those instructions. When post move-ups are begun, the activity levels of the field crews increase, and they have to be protected from high fatigue levels, both to ensure continued good patient care and to ensure their own safety. The number of 24-hour shifts will usually decrease. Sleep time also decreases; "home stations" decline in number and crews actually work many more of the hours that they are on duty. *An entire way of life is changed, and the communications personnel are perceived as the ones changing it.* If you have been newly admitted into a communications training program or your system has only recently begun implementation of these techniques, you may initially be very uncomfortable with the emotional fallout caused by this change in attitude. Prepare to be the bad guy for a while. With some hard work on your part, things will eventually normalize; they usually do.

### And It Comes Out Here!

Your position now combines all the duties of the first dispatchers, plus medical interrogation, pre-arrival instructions, system status management, resource allocation, relay of medical information, and much, much more. The nature of the medical communicator's job is supervisory. As a fully trained primary communicator, you will be expected to routinely make time-critical decisions for which there are no set rules and that require considerable use of your own judgment. You are required to function on a daily basis under extremely stressful conditions, and you are expected to consistently display cooperation and to utilize a team approach. It is now an accepted fact in our industry that the success or failure of any EMS provider frequently is dependent on the quality of personnel employed in the communications center. *Yours is the single most critical position in the organization.*

Although the responsibilities that are part of this position must never be taken lightly, you should take pride in the fact that you possess natural abilities and traits that led to your selection as a medical dispatcher or dispatch trainee. As you work, you will find that by establishing in your own system or department the procedures and general intent of the guidelines in this text, you can contribute to your department's effort to narrow the gap between communications and the field.

## OUR NEW PUBLIC IMAGE

As long as people have been employed in EMS, they have complained about the lack of respect and recognition they have received from the public in general, and from other medical professionals in particular. *We* know that as EMS workers, we are medical professionals. In the communications division of the industry, we must have special inborn talents and must acquire additional training and job skills that enable us to act as a vital link in the chain of patient care administration. Traditionally, we have all believed that the lack of recognition we have received for the service we provide was always someone else's fault or responsibility. This is a cop-out. *To be truly successful as a medical communicator, you must learn to take responsibility for your own actions.*

If a citizen calls your communications center for help and you can be heard laughing or carrying on side conversations with other employees, what impression do you suppose the caller forms? If a citizen comes to your headquarters or dispatch center and sees you with your feet up on the console or "roughhousing" with a group of field employees, just how professional do you think that person believes you to be? Every word you say and every action you take has a consequence, whether or not it is immediately obvious to you.

We are responsible for educating the public about the skills we possess and the help we provide. We are responsible for teaching our co-workers in field operations about the special talents that are required to work well as a communicator. Each time our behavior meets a high performance standard, we improve our private and public image; we take one step forward. Every time we allow ourselves the luxury of an unpleasant, inappropriate attitude or indulge in a bout of unprofessional behavior, we take two steps back.

Because "dispatcher" is still such an ambiguous word, our job title itself requires some redefinition. Therefore, we should refer to ourselves as *medical dispatchers, medical communicators,* or *system status controllers*. These job titles may have slightly different meanings in different systems. Essentially, you define your own job title. For convenience, all three terms are used interchangeably in this text.

## SPECIAL CONCENTRATION NEEDS IN THE COMMUNICATIONS CENTER

There is one single factor that will have more impact than any other on your *technical* performance as a medical communicator. During your time as a field care-giver, you have been programmed to structure your ability to *concentrate* in a certain manner. From the field side, your ability to deeply concentrate relates precisely to the chemical "rush" that you feel when you are responding to a call. There is a school of thought that believes that field employees in EMS actually develop a physical, chemical addiction to this chemical release. Since the factors that stimulate deep concentration in the dispatch center differ so completely from those in the field, you may have years of programming to overcome in order to perform the job of system status controller well.

In the field, your concentration level rises and falls with the application of a physical stimulus; your peak level of highest concentration is reached when administering hands-on care to a critical patient, or during a situation that threatens your own physical safety. Your concentration reaches its lowest point between calls, when you are at rest.

The continually demanding pace and detailed, complex nature of your job as a system status controller requires that you maintain peak concentration for much longer time periods, sometimes literally for hours without a break. The general assumption among EMS personnel, even among experienced medical dispatchers, is that most mistakes in the communications center are made when the activity level is very high, and the controllers are very busy. This is a false assumption. *More critical and potentially critical errors are made in the dispatch center when the pace is very slow than at any other time.*

Why? Does it make any sense that these seasoned communicators can deal with catastrophic situations, emotionally draining telephone contacts, multiple unit responses and zero-level coverage successfully, only to fall apart when the demand on the system slows down? In fact, if you understand the mechanics of what is happening to you, it makes perfect sense. When the pace slows, your years of programming kick in with what, in the field environment, is a very valid response to the stress of maintaining a frantically high level of activity. You relax; your reaction time slows, and you miss details. Your concentration level drops. Your listening skills temporarily deteriorate. Routine duties require deliberate effort. This is the time when dangerous errors are made in dispatch. Time-seasoned controllers experience this phenomenon more frequently than trainees, since those with experience usually do not feel the anxiety that is present during the training process.

In time, your response timing will be reprogrammed and restructured to meet the demands in the communications center. Until that happens, there are some steps you can take to protect yourself and to keep your accuracy level high.

> *First, understand the process.* It is not a failing on your part; *it is a situational disability that you must compensate for and work to overcome.* When you understand why this may happen to you, you can begin to guard against it.
>
> *Second, learn to recognize it when it begins to occur.* If your partners are having to prompt you, suggest actions to you, ask you questions about what you've done and why you've done it, and correct your mistakes, warning bells should go off in your head. Something is wrong, and your ability to concentrate is impaired.
>
> *Third, you can anticipate the process.* Anytime a break occurs in what has otherwise been a fast-paced shift, gear up to pay more attention. Compensate for the natural let-down. Usually, if you can anticipate the process, you can avoid it.
>
> *And fourth, if you realize that you are not able to concentrate completely on the job at hand, get up and walk away.* Dependence on a partner is the same in the dispatch center as it is in the field. If you are occupying a console position, your partners are counting on having your full attention, support, and assistance. If you cannot provide that to your partners, move away from the position. If you are away from the work area, your partners will no longer expect your help.

Chap. 1    *The Role of the Medical Communicator in Today's EMS System*    **15**

## SUMMARY AND REVIEW

1. What are some of the reasons for the changes in the organizational structures of EMS systems?

2. What are the major differences between old-style structures and newer, more progressive designs?

3. Try to diagram your own system's organizational structure. Can you do it? Is there a logical division of responsibility? Is there a logical progression of authority?

4. What are the newly defined job descriptions of the *system status manager* and the *communications supervisor*?

5. How is medical control achieved?

6. What changes can you think of that would improve quality or efficiency in your system?

7. Why is quality assurance so important?

8. What were some of the innovations that have helped redefine the role of the dispatcher in emergency medical service?

9. As medical communicators, do you agree that field-experienced EMS employees have advantages over lay persons?

10. What public image do EMS personnel have in your service area? What steps could you or your department take to change or improve your image? Combine those possible steps in chronological order to make a plan for your system to educate the media.

11. Who defines your role as a medical communicator? What elements do you think should be included in your job description?

12. Are the principles of system status management used in your system? If not, why not? If so, have your field employees been educated to understand those principles? Have your communicators?

13. What single factor most impacts the success or failure of the trainee in medical dispatch? Why?

14. Are more communications errors made when the activity level is very slow or very busy? Why?

15. What four steps can you take to avoid making those errors?

16. Review the general historical information provided in this chapter. Do you know how and when EMS systems developed in your state and community? A solid comprehension of past events can help you make intelligent, considered decisions about the future of your department and your system. This knowledge will also help you understand why things work the way they do in your area. What mistakes have been made in the past? If you had the opportunity, how would you correct those errors? How can your system avoid making those mistakes again?

17. Define *patient care*, *customer service*, and *customer satisfaction*. What do these terms mean? How do they differ?

18. Review the objectivity of your system and your department. Do your procedures and standards meet or exceed national standards

for patient care, medical dispatching, call prioritization, utilization of resources, and response time requirements? If not, are you taking unnecessary legal risks? Have the progress and innovations made in the communications center kept pace with those in other departments?

19. Having completed the previous steps, define some general short-term and long-term goals for yourself, your department, and your system.

# Chapter 2

# ATTITUDES AND MOTIVATION

*"Do all the good you can, In all the ways you can,
In all the places you can, At all the times you can,
To all the people you can, As long as ever you can."*
— *John Wesley, "Rules of Conduct"*

ESTABLISHING YOUR PRIORITIES

First, Last, and Always: Patient Care
and Customer Satisfaction

Say these words together several times: *"Patient care and customer satisfaction, patient care and customer satisfaction . . ."* These two phrases should be indelibly etched into your brain. Together, they define the sum total of how well you perform your job.

As a medical communicator in any system, your first responsibility and top priority will *always* be providing the highest quality patient care possible. This frequently means that, in addition to the normal processes of conducting medical interrogation, triaging information, giving pre-arrival instructions, and dispatching the appropriate unit, you will be expected to take action that, in other industries, is considered "going the extra mile"; it means making the small, thoughtful gestures that, believe it or not, will be remembered longest by both the patient and the person who calls for your help.

If you consider these actions and gestures extra effort outside the normal duties involved in working as a medical dispatcher, take time out right now to adjust your attitude. *This extra effort is very definitely part of your job.*

We are part of a service industry. We will be allowed to continue to provide our services only as long as we satisfy our customers' needs. This means not only providing excellent field care and meeting response time requirements, but also learning and using extraordinary customer service skills. Even if you work for a city service or a private provider with long-term, exclusive contracts, these needs must be addressed. Always remember that, in the long run, the citizens *do* have a choice of what entity will provide their emergency and nonemergency medical service. City governments *do* decide to change their EMS coverage from fire service to private provider systems. Privately held contracts *do* expire and become available to new bidders. If you have never lived through a provider contract change, you'll just have to trust me on this one: This is an event that you want to avoid if you can possibly do so. Also remember that providing customer satisfaction involves many elements other than good patient care.

### Providing for Field Care-Givers

Your second greatest responsibility as a medical communicator is to your system's field crews. You are responsible not only for the accurate prioritization of medical information, but also for identifying scene hazards; thus, to a degree, you are responsible for their safety. If you are acting as the radio operator, you are responsible for setting the tone for the entire work force that is exposed to radio traffic. *One person, simply by altering her or his tone of voice, can raise or lower the stress level of the entire system.* If you are acting as call-taker, you can set the tone of an entire call simply by the manner in which you answer the telephone and interact with the caller. You are responsible for correct allocation of resources, that is, making sure your field crews have what they need to function safely and efficiently.

You can also dramatically impact the *morale* of your field crews from your position in the dispatch center. If you know that a specific crew has run several calls back-to-back or a single call that may have been inordinately stressful for them, you can post them in a low-call volume area and let them rest for an hour or so, always understanding that the overall status of the system must also be considered. If a crew requests a particular posting location for a meal break, you can make every effort to accommodate them. You can maintain a supportive radio attitude even when the field crews do not. When a crew member calls control after she/he has run a particularly upsetting call, you can provide a sympathetic ear; many times, just allowing the crew member to talk about the call will help her/him to deal better with the accompanying stress.

## CONFIDENTIALITY AND INTEGRITY

*"Don't say things. What you are stands over you all the while, and thunders so that I cannot hear what you say to the contrary."*
— *Emerson, "Social Arms"*

The communications center is the central point for all communications concerning every aspect of an emergency medical system: our actions, our policies, our management, our resources, and each and every individual member of our entire work force. As medical communicators, we have the responsibility to maintain confidentiality not only for our patients, *but also for our employees.*

Working as a medical communicator, you will usually be the first to know about any major incident that affects your system. Because you will interact by telephone with those who call for help, you will be aware of details and circumstances surrounding some calls to which other persons will not have access. Because you will monitor patient reports to base station hospitals, you will be aware of details of some patients' illnesses or injuries. There is a tremendous responsibility that goes hand-in-hand with access to this type of information. Your charge is *always* to protect patient confidentiality to the fullest extent allowed by established procedures and written policies. Personal and private information is not to be communicated outside the communications center, even to other employees. Dealing with the media is a separate issue discussed elsewhere in this text.

You will also have access to a completely different type of information that is no less confidential than that already discussed . As a system status controller, you will periodically receive misdirected telephone calls and requests for messages to be relayed to your work force. You may be the first to know that one employee's electricity has been cut off for nonpayment; you may be the first to know that another is experiencing marital difficulties. It cannot be stated too often or too strongly that *this type of information is not for circulation*. ALWAYS, ALWAYS, before you speak, stop and think: If you were experiencing the same difficulties, how would you feel when you realized that the information had been circulated throughout the work force, and all of your co-workers knew of your particular situation? If information is received that causes concern about an employee's performance or ability to provide quality medical treatment, that information should be *quietly and confidentially* relayed to someone of supervisory or management rank; non-work-related, personal information received in confidence (either specifically requested or simply assumed by the other party) should not be passed on at all.

From our positions in the communications center, we have the potential to affect the attitudes of employees in field operations, maintenance, supply, and so on. Gossip, whether maliciously intended or not, is very, very strongly discouraged. If a crisis (or a perceived crisis) arises that is affecting the morale of your department or other departments, your clear duty is not to pass the information on to other employees, but to report the details as you know them immediately to a manager so that the problem can be quickly resolved. Because of the critical and confidential nature of the controller's job, failure to comply with the above stated guidelines may seriously jeopardize your continued ability to function as a medical communicator.

## MAINTAINING A POSITIVE ATTITUDE

Nobody can be "up" all the time. If you know people who always appear to be positive and never seem to feel anger or sadness, chances are that they're either very good actors, accomplished liars, or certifiably psychotic and in desperate need of being institutionalized.

Even if you greatly enjoy your job and truly believe in the philosophies of the system in which you work, there will be days when everything goes wrong. Your alarm clock didn't go off, the kids would **not** get out of bed, and you had a flat tire. You forgot to start the clothes dryer last night, and your uniform is cold and wet. The person you just relieved was out the door as soon as you were in; you have no idea what's going on in this system you're supposed to be managing. Your predecessor left the remains of last night's dinner on your dispatch console. Your supervisor just came in, looked around, and asked, "Do you live like this at home?" All the anger and frustration that normally result from these sources of stress have to go somewhere; if you keep them inside, you'll explode. The first person who tries to speak to you over the radio or who dares to dial your telephone number is going to get it *right between the eyes.*

At this point, you should already clearly understand the potential your attitude has to impact the rest of your system, your work force, and your clients (private citizens, other public service agencies, and hospital personnel). No reasonable communications supervisor will ask that you maintain a positive attitude 100 percent of the time. *Every reasonable supervisor will require that you learn and utilize voice control techniques to prevent negativity, anger, fear, or sarcasm from being evident in your voice.*

Many behavior modification and lifestyle changing techniques and options are discussed elsewhere in this text. Now all you need to know is this: When you *know* you're angry, frustrated, and out of control, what can you do *right now* to change it?

**Let go of your fantasies.** If you are employed in emergency medical service, you probably already largely define your self-image in terms of your work. Your estimation of your own worth directly relates to the job you do and how well you do it. Hand-in-hand with your agreement to perform a job function goes a set of expectations of what that job will be like. Each of us has a series of videotapes that play in our brains; I'll bet I can even tell you what's contained on yours.

> *Traffic on the dispatch channel is constant; you are alone in the dark communications center. The phones begin to ring. Grandma is having a heart attack, shootings and stabbings abound, and a busload of orphans has been involved in a major accident at the outside boundary of your service area. A neighboring community has emergency calls holding and no units available for dispatch; they scream for mutual aid. Their dispatcher is terrified, and begs for your help. You reassure her that help is on the way. Callers cry for a quick ambulance response and plead with you to tell them what to do to keep Grandma from dying. You calmly and quickly dispatch the correct units, give complicated pre-arrival instructions, and keep your documentation and post move-ups current. Field crews become impatient; they scream and snap at you on the radio. You calm them down and give them whatever information they need. When the crisis is over, many people cluster around you, jockeying for position to express their thanks. They take turns repeatedly telling you just how*

*wonderful you are. The big boss of the entire system says, "You handled that so well. I don't know what we'd do without you." You square your shoulders, put on a sunny smile, and bravely say, "It's all part of the job. Anyone could have done it."*

Oh, please. Grow up. If this seems unrealistic or foreign to you, chances are that you aren't even aware of your own fantasies. It's human nature to have them; you may think of them as expectations rather than fantasies. Whatever you choose to call them, they still exist, and they still impact your attitude. *Anything that affects your attitude will also eventually affect your tone of voice.*

Many times, our expectations grow out of simple ignorance. By nature, each human sees her/his set of circumstances, problems, or immediate job tasks as the most important in the world. If you do not understand what makes other people behave the way they do, your frustration will mount to an unacceptable level. At that point, it will be heard in your voice.

Realize that the people with whom you deal on a daily basis are probably not all bad, stupid, ignorant, evil, or conspiring together to drive you insane. They are fellow humans, and therefore are subject to the basic laws of human nature. Most people view each demand to perform as a form of attack; humans respond to attacks either by counterattacking or by escaping, through the use of an inexhaustible supply of tactics (see Figure 2.1).

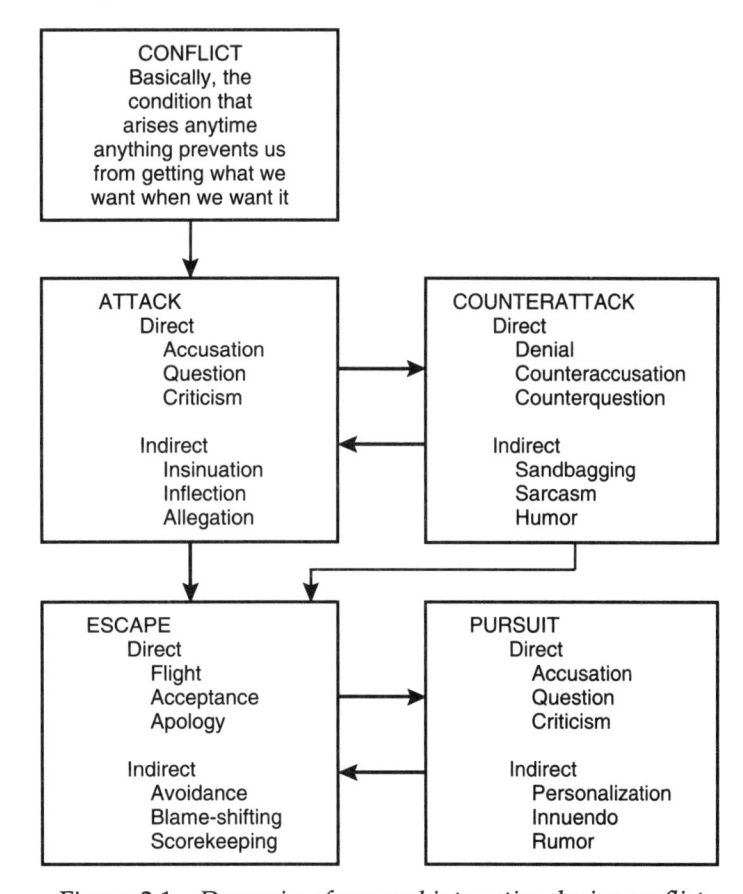

```
                    ┌─────────────────┐
                    │    CONFLICT     │
                    │  Basically, the │
                    │  condition that │
                    │  arises anytime │
                    │ anything prevents us │
                    │ from getting what we │
                    │ want when we want it │
                    └────────┬────────┘
                             │
                             ▼
        ┌─────────────────┐       ┌─────────────────┐
        │     ATTACK      │──────▶│  COUNTERATTACK  │
        │     Direct      │       │      Direct     │
        │    Accusation   │       │      Denial     │
        │    Question     │       │  Counteraccusation │
        │    Criticism    │       │  Counterquestion │
        │                 │       │                 │
        │    Indirect     │◀──────│     Indirect    │
        │   Insinuation   │       │   Sandbagging   │
        │   Inflection    │       │    Sarcasm      │
        │   Allegation    │       │     Humor       │
        └────────┬────────┘       └────────┬────────┘
                 │                         │
                 ▼                         ▼
        ┌─────────────────┐       ┌─────────────────┐
        │     ESCAPE      │──────▶│     PURSUIT     │
        │     Direct      │       │      Direct     │
        │     Flight      │       │    Accusation   │
        │   Acceptance    │       │    Question     │
        │    Apology      │       │    Criticism    │
        │                 │       │                 │
        │    Indirect     │◀──────│    Indirect     │
        │   Avoidance     │       │  Personalization │
        │  Blame-shifting │       │    Innuendo     │
        │  Scorekeeping   │       │     Rumor       │
        └─────────────────┘       └─────────────────┘
```

Figure 2.1 *Dynamics of personal interaction during conflict*

Take the time to understand the nature of the human response. Then adjust your fantasies to be more in line with realistic expectations, and reshoot your own videotape.

**Be where you are.** Unless you are trapped in a waking nightmare in which you work for what is truly *the* worst EMS system on the planet, your anger and frustrations are probably made up of many components. As you deal with crisis situations and make time-critical decisions in the communications center, other events and factors are lurking in the dark part of your brain, waiting for the chance to jump up and ruin your day. The demands of non-work-related aspects of your life don't go away when you clock in for your shift. They move into the background, rubbing their hands and smirking, knowing that their time will come.

A phenomenon frequently observed in high-stress occupations like ours is the *flash*. A controller methodically deals with truly critical situations involving life and death for hours, days, or even weeks at a time, never missing a beat. Suddenly, one innocuous comment is made, and the dispatcher literally explodes. Roll videotape.

> *Every night before you send your child to bed, you slip a PopTart into the toaster. Each morning while you dress for work, your four-year-old depresses the slide on the toaster and waits impatiently for the warm pastry to pop out. This morning, probably because she's seen those commercials on television, she manages to open the freezer door and take out a single-serving lasagna dinner. After carefully removing the wrapping, she forces the frozen block of pasta into the brand-new VCR that your spouse gave you for Christmas. The ice melts, and water and tomato sauce run into the machine. Much screaming and yelling immediately follow your discovery of this event.*
>
> *When you arrive at work, things are quiet and calm. As soon as you sit down at your console, all hell breaks loose. As you dispatch call after call, thoughts of the earlier scene at home keep popping up. Your spouse is still very angry, your child does not understand ("I saw that little boy do it on TV"), and you have no idea when you'll be able to afford to have the VCR repaired. You feel guilty where your spouse is concerned, because you should be more organized and pay more attention to what your children are doing. You feel guilty because you screamed at a four-year-old with big sad eyes who obviously didn't understand. Your life is a living hell.*
>
> *You deal well with the high activity level at work until a nurse calls from a local dialysis center. He says that, because you delayed dispatch of a scheduled patient transport to his facility, all other patients who have scheduled appointments today will now be late. He feels that your service is unsatisfactory, and that the behavior exhibited by both you and your system is extremely unprofessional.*
>
> *See Jane. See Jane flash. See Jane deliver an arrogant, self-righteous little lecture to a fellow medical professional about the nature of emergency medical service. See how Jane mistakenly believes the caller cares about what kind of day she's having. Watch as the nurse calls the system administrator to complain.*
>
> *My, my. This must be the system administrator now. He is the unhappy*

> *man with the disappointed and angry look on his face. Listen as he plays back the tape for Jane. See Jane. Jane is sad and embarrassed.*

These are facts of life: Most parents today cannot financially afford to work only in the home. Most of us never have enough time for everything we want to do. Most of us never have enough money. Most of us cannot please all the people, both at work and away, who make demands on our time. The attempt to balance the conflicting demands of home and work can be exhausting. The flash may not occur while you are at work. If you are usually structured and well disciplined, you may subconsciously delay the flash until you are in what you perceive as the less critical environment of your home. If you're having a rough shift, you can convince yourself that you don't really have *time* to vent. This very common type of stress release, and its consequences, can be avoided. *When you're at work, be at work. When you're at home, be at home.* Monitor yourself and your reactions to your work environment. If you know the potential for the flash exists, you can plan to avoid it; and when you realize it's happening, there are two things you can do *right now* to stop the process.

**Take a Deep Breath and Smile.** When you do this, you will feel two *immediate* benefits; one is emotional, and the other physical.

What does this technique accomplish, and why does it work? First, the associations that most of us have with this phrase are classic examples of *environmental programming*. How many times have you heard someone say, "Take a deep breath *and relax*". Not just, "Take a deep breath," or simply, "Relax," but "Take a deep breath *and relax*." How many times have you repeated the phrase to an emotionally distraught patient on a call, or a hysterical caller on the telephone? This is a phrase most of us have heard all our lives; each time you hear it spoken this way, the connection between the two actions is reinforced. Our minds have been programmed by our environments (by people, the printed word, radio, and television) to understand that the two activities are connected, or that one causes the other. Even when you only repeat part of the phrase to yourself, your brain will subconsciously supply the other part.

Second, there is an immediate physical benefit. When you take a very deep breath, the muscles in your neck, back, and chest wall contract. The natural reaction to the contraction of a set of muscles is a relaxation of the same muscles. It's the body's way of normalizing. (If our bodies didn't automatically do this, we would forget until we wound up like springs, folded in on ourselves, and bounced uncontrollably around the room.) It's hard to sound pleasant when you feel tense; it's much easier when you *relax*.

After you have taken the deep breath, and *before you open your mouth to speak, smile.* As is discussed in the Communications sections of this text, it is virtually impossible to invest your voice with one emotion while there is another showing on your face. Say a phrase while you frown. Now smile and say it again. Can you hear the difference? When you smile, the shape of the sound wave created when you speak subtly changes. *When you smile with your face, your listener will hear the smile in your voice.* You will have mastered a difficult situation, and effectively "turned the other cheek." This intervention technique will not only prevent you from making a serious error in judgment, but will also give you the opportunity to feel amazingly smug and self-righteous about your behavior in contrast to that of others. Allow yourself to slide down and wallow in that feeling for a few minutes. It's not going to hurt you.

Some of the most dramatic improvements I have seen during voice control training have come about because the trainee took a deep breath and smiled.

In the long run, your ability to provide customer satisfaction will improve in direct relationship with your ability to maintain a positive attitude, to control flash reactions, and to control your voice.

## SUMMARY AND REVIEW

1. What is your first priority as a medical communicator?

2. What is your second priority?

3. What practical ways can you think of to help you positively impact the morale of your field employees? Can any of these steps be written into policy or procedure for the medical communicators in your system?

4. What relationship does the medical dispatcher have to the process of maintaining confidentiality for the patient? For the field employee?

5. Do you know what's on your videotape titled, "My Work In Medical Communications"?

6. What is a flash?

7. What are four ways to stop yourself when you begin to flash? What are the benefits of each technique?

*Chapter* **3**

# THE OPERATION OF THE COMMUNICATIONS CENTER

*"The key to getting ahead is setting aside
eight hours a day for work and eight hours
a day for sleep .... and making sure they're not the same hours."*
— *Gene Brown, in the Danbury, Connecticut News-Times*

SETTING YOURSELF UP TO WIN

When you design or redesign a communications department, you should do just that: *design* it. Think about what you are doing. Even in the face of what appears to be insurmountable opposition, you can literally set yourself up to win by following these seven simple steps:

1. *Believe in yourself.* There is a great difference between believing that a thing is true, hoping that it's true, and knowing it's true. Know, before you start, that you can accomplish anything you set out to do. You already have several factors on your side. First, you have identified various areas where your system needs improvement; otherwise, you would not be reading this text. Realizing that improvement *can be made* is half the battle. Second, you are already motivated to attempt to change things; again, if you weren't, you wouldn't be wasting your time here. And third, you should realize that many people in systems all over the country have faced the same stumbling blocks and the same challenges that you face now, and have achieved success.

2. *Think of yourself as creative.* Creativity is viewed by many people as a magical quality possessed only by a lucky few. We have been led to believe that most of our natural creative talent was systematically destroyed when we were children. "I can't draw," you say. "I can't sing. I don't have a creative or artistic bone in my body."

So what? Most ideas that seem truly inspired can be reduced to simple logic. For example, take a young man named Nolan Bushnell. He watched people and observed that people like to play games, and that they like to watch television. How, he asked himself, could he combine the two to invent a new form of amusement? The resulting invention, the first Atari video game, turned into a hundred-million-dollar industry. Dismantle the walls you've built to protect yourself and let your mind go. And, remember . . . the more often you engage in creative problemsolving, the easier it gets.

3. *Break out of your patterns.* Humans learn by following a simple pattern: remember what works. It's this process that keeps us from having to rediscover fire each time we want to boil water for tea. Sometimes, however, we allow ourselves to see only what's been tried before. Discover a new angle, paint a new picture, try a different approach. Learn to think in terms of, "What if we did this?"

4. *Don't stop learning.* When you get stuck, change your environment, look at things from another person's point of view, dig until you find some new research material. While information specific to EMS may not always be available, there are still hundreds of thousands of sources for information about people, psychology, equipment, and so on. Learn something new, and then relate that knowledge to what you're trying to accomplish.

5. *Allow yourself room to make adjustments.* Don't commit yourself so firmly to one idea or one plan of action that you can't change gears if another, better idea comes along. If your first plan doesn't work exactly the way you imagined, it's not necessarily *wrong;* it may just need some fine-tuning, or a more satisfactory option may just have become available for the first time.

6. *Find the second "right" answer.* Many times, the best solution to a problem is not the most obvious one. We are conditioned by our culture to place values on things or ideas in terms of black and white, good and bad, right and wrong. Broaden your perspective and learn to see things as they relate to each other. List several possible solutions and then debate them with yourself or others. How would you "sell" a particular idea? When you list the advantages and disadvantages of any plan, the definitive characteristics will become more clear to you.

7. *Ask yourself this question: "What is it like to work with me?"* Sometimes the one thing that blocks effective action is the attitude of the person trying to take that action. A field paramedic may have excellent technical skills in starting IVs; however, if his attitude so angers the patient and family that they refuse to let him initiate treatment, then of what use will those skills be? Evaluate your own "people" skills; be sure that lack of expertise in communicating with people is not what's holding your program back.

## THE LOCATION OF THE COMMUNICATIONS CENTER

Some years ago, someone said, "Communications should be separated from operations." Systems all over the country took steps to isolate their dispatch personnel in different buildings, and sometimes even in completely different parts of the service area than those used as bases by the system's field crews.

Time has proven that, in most instances, this was not a good idea. When dispatch personnel are separated from the field crews with whom they work, they become stale. The system's most vital links are forced to work in a vacuum. Funny things happen in vacuums; we lose our perspective, and small things get blown completely out of proportion into large, unmanageable things.

I believe what was originally meant by that statement was something entirely different. I believe that the statement was intended to mean that production managers and field supervisors should not *supervise* communications personnel. *Experienced communicators should supervise communications personnel.* One of the most frequently heard complaints about managers is, "She thinks she can tell me what to do, but she couldn't sit here and do my job on a bet." The effective manager leads by example, and so must possess all the skills her/his line employees use every day.

Positioning the control center in or near the field headquarters building brings many benefits. Communications personnel are kept better informed. They are more easily motivated, since they are made to feel involved with the overall operation of the system. By observing each other closely as their work is accomplished, field and communications personnel can give each other valuable insights and suggestions for improvement. And small problems with or questions from field personnel can be resolved at the end of each shift, rather than being allowed to build up for months at a time.

## DESIGNING THE PHYSICAL LAYOUT

The most important single factor to remember when designing the physical "plant" of the communications center is to *consult the people who will work there.* Many times, this valuable source of ideas is overlooked in favor of the experts, who not only don't know how the medical communicator's job is performed, but who won't have to live with the consequences of their design.

The physical environment of any group of employees can dramatically impact their ability to perform their jobs well. Communicators in many systems have to sit at their consoles for 12 hours at a time. An improperly constructed chair that does not provide lumbar support can cause crippling back pain; discomfort of any kind interferes with your ability to concentrate.

Temperature is important; if it is too hot or too cold, the dispatcher's thoughts may naturally focus on the environmental discomfort instead of the details of the task at hand. Temperature controls should be placed where the controllers can easily access them.

Lighting is another critical concern. Bright overhead fluorescent lighting can cause serious eye strain, which again can impair job performance. Lower lighting levels achieved through the use of incandescent fixtures can lower stress levels overall.

What will happen if power is lost to your building? What will be your auxiliary power supply? What about the equipment necessary for dispatch? Where will you position it?

Gather together the personnel who will be working in the communications center; invite them to brainstorm with you to help identify all the elements involved in the design. Have the controllers walk through the steps required to perform their jobs. How can you place the equipment to minimize the amount of physical stress involved in using it? What kind of soundproofing precautions should be taken? Should the control center be in a secured area? How will you secure it? What if you moved this console here, or there? How will this look in six months? What if, what if, what if?

Write down every idea and every suggestion. Fine-tune the plan and check out the practicalities of putting the ideas into practice. Then get together for another round of planning.

During this type of design process, no idea should ever be dismissed out-of-hand as silly or inappropriate. If one person verbalizes an opinion or a concern, chances are that two others are thinking it. For a design process to be successful, planning must be accomplished to address every opinion, every concern, and every eventuality.

## SETTING DEPARTMENTAL STANDARDS

Who will ultimately define the medical communicator's job? *You will, by the standards you set for yourself and others, and the way you conduct yourself each shift that you work.* Remember two things: First, that people tend to become what we expect them to be; and second, that we get in life exactly what we will take, no more and no less. If you expect and accept nothing but the best from yourself and your department, the best is exactly what you will get.

The first step toward establishing a standard level of performance is to set basic requirements for hiring new trainees. What should these prerequisites be for your department? It depends on the type of system you work in and what your end goals are. In my system, each applicant to the communications training program must have achieved paramedic certification, must have worked in some capacity in the system for a minimum of six continuous months just prior to the training start date, and must currently be certified to provide basic life support (CPR). Your hiring prerequisites may be more or less stringent in the beginning; you may choose to change or upgrade them at a later time.

You should be aware of one major consideration before you set your hiring standards: Field personnel who work in emergency medical service may not respect those who are not medically trained. You can disagree with this point until the world looks level, and that won't change the fact that in many systems it's true. The reasons why it's true are not bad; instead, they are realistic and healthy.

Field paramedics and emergency medical technicians *know* they're special people. They can do things that those in other professions can't do; they can handle more, they can stay calm longer. They routinely work under the worst imaginable conditions. They directly confront pain and suffering, death and dying day after day. Field EMS workers perform highly skilled tasks in the dark, in extreme temperatures, during severe storms, and frequently in the immediate area where violent crimes have taken place and may occur again. They are stronger, both physically and emotionally, than other people. Even hospital personnel don't have to deal with situations as critical and uncontrolled as those field care-givers regularly face; our field crews usually have things "cleaned up" by the time they turn their patients over to emergency room employees.

Probably the most important personality trait of the outstanding field care-giver is her/his independence. This quality is fostered and nurtured in field employees; out on the street, they usually can't turn to someone else for advice or expect someone else to shoulder responsibility. They're on their own, and they know it. This independence makes it extremely difficult for field workers to accept arbitrary direction, especially when it comes from someone trained to a lower level of expertise than they. One of the few situations where this equal or higher training level may not be required can exist in a system where specific communicators have been in place for long periods of time, and have proven themselves to excel at their jobs. Specific dispatch training and demonstrated skills may replace medical certifications; however, establishing the credibility of a dispatch professional without medical training equal to that of field employees takes time, effort, and patience.

In most systems, especially newer ones, a clearly defined and accepted level of medical skill must exist on the part of communicators, and a considerable amount of respect and authority must be granted to them, before they will be able to successfully perform all their job duties in any EMS response system. *This maximum use of available talent can only come about when medical communicators are trained to meet or exceed the certification requirements of the highest certification level in the field.*

What about continuing performance standards? If you use a computer-assisted dispatch system, shouldn't communicators in your system be able to type a certain number of words per minute? How many? Is there a level of typing skill below which the dispatcher's job performance is less than satisfactory?

When you begin administering regularly scheduled written examinations to communications personnel, what will be a passing score? Should those standards become tougher as time in a position increases? Also consider standards for conduct, dress, attendance, and punctuality.

Sometimes, the most important thing about a decision is to make it. The important point here is to begin somewhere, standardize the procedures, have demanding but reasonable expectations, allow room to upgrade and improve, document the rules and requirements, *and then stick with the plan.*

## PROTECTING YOUR POSITION

When you have reached a decision about departmental standards at entry level and above, you and all communications personnel must adhere to them *without exception.*

If you allow field personnel who are injured and on light duty to automatically be reassigned to the communications center, you are creating an image in the minds of other system employees (The Home for Aged and Infirm Paramedics). If you allow an SSC who is having emotional problems to function, even temporarily, at a standard lower than her/his colleagues, you again create an image in the minds of others. If an insulin-dependent field medic is considered too unstable to continue working in the field, does it make any sense at all to place that person in the communications department? Well, of course it doesn't. Since the medical dispatcher's function has traditionally been viewed as less work and less stressful than the field environment, managers of other departments sometimes reassign employees to the dispatch center as "favors." Although practices like these have gone on for years, they are *not* the result of rational, logical thinking. They are the result of following the path of least resistance; they are in place because "We've always done it this way."

The medical dispatcher's job is at least as critical as that of the field care-giver. You must protect the quality and integrity of your position by refusing to allow your department to be used as a dumping ground for any other department in the system.

## TYPES OF PERSONALITIES IN THE COMMUNICATIONS CENTER

As any team of medical dispatchers settles in, expands their scope of responsibility, increases in number, and spends time in place on the job, the development of certain distinct personality types will be observed. Each communicator may possess characteristics of several different types. Some personality types possess largely positive qualities, and some chiefly negative.

The ultimate goal of each medical communicator and each communications department must be to strike a balance between technical and mechanical skills and people management skills.

Review the following personality profiles. How would you categorize your co-workers? Which qualities do you recognize in yourself?

**The Parent.** The parent is a "natural" in the newly defined role of the medical communicator. She/he is a born nurturer, and cares a great deal about people. The parent has the inborn ability to perform many tasks at once, and naturally strikes a balance between technical excellence and the human needs of customers, field personnel, and co-communicators.

The parent quickly forms a symbiotic relationship with all the other personality types in the control center. Frequently, other dispatchers and field personnel discuss details of their personal lives or their emotional responses to their jobs with the parent, seeking advice or guidance. The parent, whether she or he realizes it consciously, enjoys and encourages this dependence from colleagues. The parent personality feels compelled to "fix" things. When problems cannot be quickly resolved at the parent's level, guilt, frustration, and feelings of failure result. The parent also brings a great deal of emotional investment to the job. This investment, combined with the strain of emotional over-involvement with co-workers, can add up to more baggage than one person can carry.

The parent, for the same reasons that she/he is so good at the medical communicator's job, is at high risk for emotional overload. Conversely, the *balanced* parent personality is the type most likely to survive long-term employment as a medical dispatcher while maintaining a healthy mental and emotional perspective.

**The Child.** The child is usually bright, and learns quickly. Technical excellence is rapidly achieved. Judgment (when not impaired by sulking, temper tantrums, or a refusal to exercise any judgment at all in order to prove a point) is usually rational and sound. However, of all the personality types observed in career communicators, the child has the poorest chance of retaining her or his employment.

The child is insecure on a very basic level, and has a negative self-image. To counteract her/his feelings of inadequacy, the child requires almost constant attention. When "good" or positive attention is not available, "bad" attention or feedback will serve to satisfy the child's needs.

This personality will experience a continuing series of personal disasters and will openly discuss these problems with anyone who makes even a pretense of listening. Illnesses and injuries, whether real or imagined, will occur with regularity. It is not uncommon to find the child's personnel file filled with the documentation of disciplinary actions, all for the same infraction repeated over and over. The same complaints about the child will be made by her/his co-workers again and again. Identical, multiple counseling sessions between the supervisor and the employee will recur, and still the inappropriate behavior will continue. There is, however, always one qualifying factor: none of the problems just discussed will be the child's fault.

Allowing one employee to perform to a standard below that of all others is unfair to the remainder of the work force; it is also dangerous. Without radical modification of the child's behavior, the probability is very high that this communicator's employment will be involuntarily terminated. The employee will be fired not for lack of job skills, but for repeatedly committing "small" errors: habitual tardiness, failure to report for her/his shift in uniform, or a refusal to comply with a routine policy or procedure. The termination, while unavoidable from a departmental or other managerial standpoint, will be tragic in one sense: a great deal of rare talent will be wasted, simply because the communicator failed to recognize inappropriate behavior patterns, or failed to change them.

**The Scorekeeper.** This personality type keeps score in relationships. The scorekeeper carries in her/his head, consciously or unconsciously, a mental ledger in which she/he constantly records numbers and events.

Scorekeepers record, by some numerical system all their own, how much work they have produced in comparison with their co-workers; obviously, the scorekeeper always contributes more. They note the numbers of positive and negative comments made both to themselves and to others; the resulting totals lead them to feel either picked on or vastly superior to others. They rate the emotional support they give to their partners, and compare it to that which they receive in return. They keep a running inventory of all the mean or unkind things that have been done to them. They even tally how much attention they receive from co-workers and supervisors, and almost always come up wanting.

The result of most scorekeeping is that the person involved in the practice ends up feeling that she/he has done more, worked harder, given more, and has received substantially less in return. These feelings build exponentially to dissatisfaction, deprivation, anger and resentment. Scorekeepers generally deal with these negative feelings in one of two ways. Some try to correct the imbalance by stopping the giving process cold, that is "I'm not doing anything else for him until he does something for me," or "I'm not doing any more work until she does her share." Very rarely does this strategy work; it almost invariably backfires. The reason for the failure is this: Those people who automatically give to and do for others are also often the "idea people" or the initiators in a relationship. When the scorekeeper decides to stop the process, the person with whom the conflict exists often does nothing. The scale is not balanced. The scorekeeper, who is often by nature compulsive and a perfectionist, must watch in mounting frustration, anger, and resentment while absolutely nothing gets done.

Another method used by scorekeepers is to assume the role of the martyr. No matter how much the other person doesn't do or fails to contribute, the scorekeeper continues to do more than her/his share. She or he never verbally addresses the problem or the negative feelings accompanying it. When the scorekeeper has no more to give, she/he explodes or flashes, displaying an obviously inappropriate emotional response. This is categorically unfair to the other party or parties involved, since either they are unaware of the scorekeeper's standards for giving, or the standards are extreme and unrealistic.

A different but related aspect of this personality type can be seen in the "I'll do it" manifestation. In this case, the scorekeeper has already tallied the score and found the partner or colleague wanting.

Therefore, again without ever verbally and honestly expressing dissatisfaction, she or he simply performs every required task alone. These people can be truly fascinating to watch. They can solicit and input call information, dispatch the emergency response, give pre-arrival instructions, provide crews with additional information, and answer several auxiliary telephone lines all at once. Although this activity can demonstrate their considerable technical skills, it also paints a picture of very poor mental and emotional health.

While scorekeepers view themselves as imminently competent, highly skilled professionals who must constantly take up the slack for their lesser-qualified co-workers, they are invariably seen in a different light by their colleagues. Partners complain that the scorekeepers with whom they work are bossy, nosy, controlling, and short-tempered.

Scorekeeping is learned behavior. A certain amount of scorekeeping is normal; it is a natural self-protective mechanism used to keep the scales from becoming too out of balance. However, some people practice scorekeeping to an excessive degree. These are usually people who believe that they are not worthy of and will never receive admiration and respect from their co-workers. Scorekeeping essentially and invariably develops secondary to a negative self-image; it is a subliminal attempt to change that image to a positive one.

The first step in modifying a behavior pattern is recognizing that the pattern exists. Many such patterns are developed in childhood, and as such, are not anyone's fault. However, some planned emotional investment will be necessary to break these habits. If you have recognized this pattern in your own behavior, you must begin to change it. If you are regularly feeling, "I give so much, and get so little in return," or "The work would never get done if I didn't do it," then you must learn to tell your co-workers how you feel. Other people cannot read your mind, or know instinctively what your needs and wants are. Even if they could, it is not their responsibility to do so. Also, it is important to remember that each individual is just that: an individual. Your co-workers were brought up in environments different than yours; they learned different standards for acceptable behavior. In addition, there are many people who reach chronological maturity without ever knowing clearly what the rules are. Your responsibility is to tell your partners what your expectations are, clearly and without emotional conditions.

When scorekeepers begin the attempt to change their behavior patterns, they tell the offending partner what their expectations are. This almost never accomplishes its intended purpose with the first attempt. The typical reaction of the scorekeeper is, "Well, I tried it, and it didn't work." It is important to understand that behavior modification is a process, not an event. If you are a scorekeeper, you must make the commitment to dedicate to the problem whatever time, effort, and number of attempts are required to resolve it. You *can* resolve this problem, and change the unhappy situation into a happy one. Just don't give up.

**The Tattletale.** The tattletale, like the child, suffers from low self-esteem. As a result, she or he demands attention. Although tattletales are usually highly skilled, they do not view personal accomplishments and competency levels realistically. Both in an attempt to make their own actions appear more satisfactory, and to draw attention to real or imagined abuses, tattletales point out the "flaws" in their colleagues' attitudes and performance.

The tattletale's actions may take one of two general forms: she or he may report errors, large or small, clearly defined or open to interpretation, committed by other communicators. In its most insidious, most destructive form, the tattletale syndrome may manifest itself in the employee's persistent habit of repeating casual or maliciously intended comments or gossip. The tattletale will repeat hurtful statements to the person about whom they were made, usually under the guise of friendship: "I'm telling you this because I think you should know," or "If he said that about me, I'd want to be told." While the tattletale's methods of gaining attention usually do not interfere with the actual performance of her/his job duties, they do accomplish one unfortunate result: the tattletale's actions almost never pass unnoticed or unidentified by other workers. The tattletale rapidly loses the trust and respect of fellow communicators, supervisors, and field personnel. When tattletale behavior is obvious and frequently repeated, this lack of trust can prove to be crippling to the communicator involved.

**The Competitor.** The competitor sees every job task or situation as a contest, a race, or a measurement of skill or dedication. This personality constantly seeks perfection in her or his own performance, and constantly finds that performance lacking. Because of the dissatisfaction that results, competitors continuously strive to prove that their skills and knowledge are superior to others: "I know the service area better than he does," or "I can do the job faster and more accurately than she can." They see all other employees as adversaries.

A degree of healthy, friendly competition should be encouraged in any quality-conscious communications center. Through supportive competition, the learning process for communicators is facilitated. However, when an individual's competitive spirit accelerates to a high level, personal conflicts can quickly take precedence over the knowledge gained. Super-competitive behavior is usually viewed by other medical dispatchers as an attack, and will be responded to accordingly.

**The Rock.** The rock is usually a positive person by nature. Rocks require a high standard of performance from themselves, while remaining supportive in the face of substandard performance by others.

The rock remains calm, even placid, in unpleasant situations and crises. When problems arise, the rock is patient and content to request resolution through routine channels. She/he rarely displays bad temper, appearing "unflappable" under even the worst of circumstances. This communicator inspires a high degree of confidence and comfort among co-workers; colleagues and field employees alike feel safe when the rock is on duty. Supervisory personnel rely on their rocks to provide honest, fair evaluations of other communicators, and to relay their perceptions of departmentwide efficiency, job satisfaction, and so on.

The rock is an authority figure to other SSCs, and relishes both the responsibilities attendant with that authority and the satisfaction derived from dealing well with a variety of difficult situations. Frequently, these medical communicators believe that to discuss transient personal feelings of frustration or failure (which are inevitable in this job) is to admit weakness. They are so committed to successfully handling the problems of others and still remaining in control that they cannot afford to stop and deal with their own emotional difficulties.

This personality is at the highest risk for emotional overload and/or damage as a medical communicator. If you can identify in yourself some of the primary qualities of the rock, you must constantly monitor your own stress level and allow yourself to vent appropriately.

## SCHEDULING AND STAFFING

In many systems across the country, communications personnel are avid proponents of the principles of system status management. They use it every day, and they know it works. System status managers routinely grind out the numbers that tell them how many units must be on the street at any given hour to handle the historical call demand. These systems regularly meet their response time requirements, their unit deployment plans are realistic and flexible, and their overall level of care is high. Their field employees are satisfied with the demands made on them by the system, their customers and clients are happy with the level of customer satisfaction that is delivered, *and their communications personnel are nuts*. Why? Because they forgot to implement the principles of system status management in their own departments.

In the beginning, you may only have one dispatcher on duty all the time. This is usually unsatisfactory, since it severely limits the abilities of the SSC to give complicated or lengthy pre-arrival instructions. However, in many systems, at least in the early stages of operation, it is a financial necessity.

As the demands on the system increase, the system status manager will evaluate and re-evaluate the need for unit hours on the street. The supply (field unit hours) must always meet or exceed the demand (number of calls run in any hour). *Each time demand is calculated for the field side, increases in demand should also be recognized in the communications center.*

Spend a day or a week observing in your dispatch center. How many telephone calls are made for each ambulance response? While most of us would immediately assume that in a competent system, one phone call should equal one response, this is usually just not so. *At least* two telephone calls are usually required to complete one ambulance response. Emergency responses may require calling back several times to elicit additional information or to give continuing pre-arrival instructions. Nonemergency transports may require five or six calls to coordinate the event among all the parties concerned. Add to these calls the number of billing queries, information requests, and administrative calls processed in your communications center each day, and the number will surprise you.

If you have two communicators on duty at all times, one should ideally answer the telephones while the other handles the radio traffic. If one controller is responsible for all the incoming telephone calls, how often is she or he actually answering the phone? Take the number of hours in the dispatcher's shift, subtract time for meals and breaks, and identify the amount of time the employee is actually expected to be in position and working. Convert hours to minutes by multiplying by 60. Now divide the number of available minutes in the controller's shift by the number of incoming phone calls expected in the shift. *In some systems, this initial evaluation reveals that the communicator is expected to begin dealing with a new caller once every one to three minutes throughout the shift.*

Get a clue. It's virtually impossible to maintain any kind of high performance standard when the activity level is constantly this high. When are these people supposed to eat? When can they go to the bathroom? The same system status management principles that protect field personnel from high fatigue levels and provide even distribution of the work load must be utilized in the dispatch center as well as in field operations.

## Structuring the Hours

The first obvious need in any communications center is to have 24-hour dispatching capabilities. At least one person must be on duty 24 hours a day. Core shifts in 8- or 12-hour increments are suggested. For example, some systems schedule four basic 12-hour shifts. Employees work from 0600 to 1800, or from 1800 to 0600; their work days are either Sunday, Monday, Tuesday and every other Wednesday, or Thursday, Friday, Saturday and every other Wednesday (see Figures 3.1a and 3.1b). In other systems, the communicators prefer to work four days on and then have four days off. Establish your core shifts, and then recalculate the demand on the system.

When demand and the amount of revenue being generated indicate an additional need, you may add a second dispatcher to the 24-hour schedule. Shift days and hours will be identical to the original schedule; now, you have two dispatchers on duty 24 hours a day. Re-evaluate system demand again.

The next step is usually to add a "power shift" to help during the busiest times. Depending on the type of service you provide, these peak demand hours may be 0900–1700, Monday through Friday (due to nonemergency call volume and administrative telephone calls), or 1700–0200, any day during the week (due to requests for emergency service). Additional shifts may be added on weekends. There are no time requirements for the number of hours any shift must work; you could add a 4-hour power shift on Saturday afternoon, or schedule a

Week 1: Employees 1, 2, 3, and 4 work Wednesday; Training shifts may be added as needed.

| | Sunday | Monday | Tuesday | Wednesday | Thursday | Friday | Saturday |
|---|---|---|---|---|---|---|---|
| Employee 1 | 0600-1800 | 0600-1800 | 0600-1800 | 0600-1800 | | | |
| Employee 2 | 0600-1800 | 0600-1800 | 0600-1800 | 0600-1800 | | | |
| Employee 3 | 1800-0600 | 1800-0600 | 1800-0600 | 1800-0600 | | | |
| Employee 4 | 1800-0600 | 1800-0600 | 1800-0600 | 1800-0600 | | | |
| Employee 5 | | | | | 0600-1800 | 0600-1800 | 0600-1800 |
| Employee 6 | | | | | 0600-1800 | 0600-1800 | 0600-1800 |
| Employee 7 | | | | | 1800-0600 | 1800-0600 | 1800-0600 |
| Alternate 1 | | | | | 1800-0600 | 1800-0600 | |
| Alternate 2 | | | | | | | 1800-0600 |
| Alternate 3 | | | | | | | |
| Employee 8 | | 0900-1700 | 0900-1700 | 0900-1700 | 0900-1700 | 0900-1700 | |
| Employee 9 | | 1700-0100 | 1700-0100 | 1700-0100 | 1700-0100 | 1700-0100 | |
| Alternate 4 | 1400-0200 | | | | | | |
| Alternate 5 | | | | | | | 1500-0300 |
| Employee 10 | | 0900-1700 | 0900-1700 | 0900-1700 | 0900-1700 | 0900-1700 | |
| Dep't. Manager | | 1000-2000 | 0800-1800 | | 1000-2000 | 0700-1700 | |
| Ass't. Manager | | | | 1200-2000 | 1200-2000 | 1200-2000 | 1200-2000 |

Figure 3.1a  *Sample communications center schedule, week 1*

Week 2: Employees 5, 6, 7, and Alternate 1 work Wednesday; Training shifts may be added as needed.

| | Sunday | Monday | Tuesday | Wednesday | Thursday | Friday | Saturday |
|---|---|---|---|---|---|---|---|
| Employee 1 | 0600-1800 | 0600-1800 | 0600-1800 | | | | |
| Employee 2 | 0600-1800 | 0600-1800 | 0600-1800 | | | | |
| Employee 3 | 1800-0600 | 1800-0600 | 1800-0600 | | | | |
| Employee 4 | 1800-0600 | 1800-0600 | 1800-0600 | | | | |
| Employee 5 | | | | 0600-1800 | 0600-1800 | 0600-1800 | 0600-1800 |
| Employee 6 | | | | 0600-1800 | 0600-1800 | 0600-1800 | 0600-1800 |
| Employee 7 | | | | 1800-0600 | 1800-0600 | 1800-0600 | 1800-0600 |
| Alternate 1 | | | | 1800-0600 | 1800-0600 | | |
| Alternate 2 | | | | | | 1800-0600 | |
| Alternate 3 | | | | | | | 1800-0600 |
| Employee 8 | | 0900-1700 | 0900-1700 | 0900-1700 | 0900-1700 | 0900-1700 | |
| Employee 9 | | 1700-0100 | 1700-0100 | 1700-0100 | 1700-0100 | 1700-0100 | |
| Alternate 4 | 1400-0200 | | | | | | |
| Alternate 5 | | | | | | | 1500-0300 |
| Employee 10 | | 0900-1700 | 0900-1700 | 0900-1700 | 0900-1700 | 0900-1700 | |
| Dep't. Manager | | 1000-2000 | 0800-1800 | | 1000-2000 | 0700-1700 | |
| Ass't. Manager | | | | 1200-2000 | 1200-2000 | 1200-2000 | 1200-2000 |

Figure 3.1b  *Sample communications center schedule, week 2*

third or fourth person to help out during the busiest hours on Monday morning.

When building your scheduling structure, remember these simple steps:

- Continue to re-examine and re-evaluate the demands on the system.
- Remember to include the communications center as a functional part of that system.
- Allow time for breaks.
- Make sure that supply (scheduled hours in the communications center) meets or exceeds the demand.
- Break out of your patterns and allow yourself to see all the possibilities for communications schedules.

Alternates versus Full-Time Communicators

Even after your system's busiest hours and communications core shifts have been established, there will be an additional staffing need in your department. Full-time employees do get sick and take vacation time. Reliable resources must be identified and trained as relief personnel. I recommend employing field personnel for this purpose. These are some of the advantages in maintaining a large pool of alternate controllers:

- They provide an easily accessible source when full-time SSCs are ill or vacationing.
- The alternate's understanding of overall system operation is increased.
- Full-time dispatchers are reminded of field concerns and attitudes; field-oriented alternates can help you to maintain a broader, more appropriate perspective.
- Alternates provide an excellent resource for short- notice overtime in the communications department.
- Employing full-time field personnel in the control center increases employee involvement and encourages interaction between operations and communications.

When training and assigning full-time field personnel in the dispatch center, you must remember one thing: *There cannot be two performance standards in a communications department.* Even though to achieve excellence, a larger time investment will be required of the alternate, her or his performance must be evaluated by the same standards as are utilized with full-time communications personnel.

## ROTATING THROUGH THE POSITIONS

In a communications center that staffs two or more dispatchers concurrently, different console positions are usually designated to fulfill specified tasks. One position may be routinely identified as that of primary call-taker and one as radio operator, for example. I strongly recommend that you limit the amount of consecutive time each communicator spends in each position. There are two reasons for this suggestion:

First, the physical act of getting up and moving to another position changes your mind-set and allows for more complete concentration. If a dispatcher is allowed to remain in one position, performing one primary function, for her or his entire shift, boredom sets in within a short time, and the communicator may begin to function on "automatic pilot." This is an extremely dangerous situation, since increased boredom and fatigue levels lead directly to errors.

Second, a preference for one position over another usually indicates both a specific strength and a weakness. Very few of us dislike doing something we're good at. If Roger hates to sit in the call-taker's position, it's probably because his stress level increases when he's working there. If he's stressed in the position, it's probably because Roger's call-taking and people management skills need improvement. Weak skills or skills needing some improvement should not be ignored or hidden, but should be identified. Retraining and practice will bring the skill levels in question up to a standard where the communicator can relax in any console position and be comfortable.

## COOPERATION

It is understood that the system status controller's job is, by nature, extremely stressful. It is also understood that you, as a medical dispatcher, can and will be affected by stresses in your personal life. Each controller is an individual and is entitled to her/his own opinions and viewpoints. However, again because of the critical nature of the controller's job and because of the close quarters in which we work, cooperation between shift partners is essential. We must help each other and support each other. Each controller must carry her/his appropriate share of the shift work load.

When a problem in cooperation between shift partners in the dispatch center is observed or reported, the first attempt to address the problem should, by all rights, be made by the shift partners themselves. Mutual agreement by all partners on a shift to foster open communication is usually the most effective approach to take. If the problem cannot be resolved by the shift partners themselves, the communications manager must resolve the situation. Again, open communication and frequent supervisory feedback are the preferred ways to resolve the problem. Shift reassignments should be made as a last resort.

## PRACTICAL PROBLEM SOLVING: WHERE'S YOUR SENSE OF HUMOR?

When you encounter a recurring problem with a communications partner, the single most important thing to remember is to maintain a sense of humor. If you can't solve whatever problem your partner is having, at least have some fun with it. For example:

> *You're working with partners who are unpleasant, aggressive, condescending, and overbearing. They insist on treating you as if you don't have a brain in your head, and constantly tell you what to do. You've given them hints all shift that they're being obnoxious, but they haven't caught on yet. Your supervisor is out of the office, so you can't resolve this problem immediately. What can you do to keep from losing your mind before your shift is over?*
>
> *Wait until the activity level in the dispatch center is fairly busy. Now move quietly up behind them. Softly hum an appropriate tune, such as the theme song from "Mr. Ed" or "If I Only Had a Brain" from The Wizard of Oz. Stop before you completely finish the song. Now move back to your console and wait.*
>
> *Within a matter of minutes, these people who have driven you crazy for hours will have that catchy little tune stuck in their heads. They will hum, they will whistle, they will tap their feet in time with the music. They'll wonder where they heard that song, and what it is. Only you will know, and you will laugh for a long, long time.*

Periodically, my own system's communicators choose to remind me who is actually in charge. Our communications center is located in a very large room, along with fire department dispatchers for our most populous client city. The telephone lines for ambulance service ring with a different type of bell than the fire department phones; our lines have a very distinctive sound. My office is about 20 feet from the controllers' work area. The backs of the dispatch consoles point toward me. Although I can't always *see* everything that is taking place in the work area, the acoustics of the building are such that I can *hear* every sound.

On a recent Monday afternoon, call volume suddenly dropped, and the medical communicators got bored. I was in my office, frantically working to meet a deadline and having completely lost my sense of humor, when I heard our console phones begin to ring. I counted two rings, and then three; I stood up and stepped to my office door. As I looked over the tops of our dispatch consoles, I suddenly realized I could see the top of only one dispatcher's head. *As the phones continued to ring, I heard this communicator say the phrase that we use to answer emergency lines.*

I vaulted over my high-backed office chair and a typing table, and headed for the work area at a dead run, screaming, *"Was that an emergency phone line? Where is everybody? Are you all by yourself out here?"* As I swung around the end console, I saw all five communicators on duty huddled on the floor in hysterics. They had used one nonemergency telephone line to dial another, let it ring for some time, and then answered as if it was an incoming emergency call. When I realized what they had done, I laughed until I cried. This little episode changed my attitude for the rest of the afternoon.

## SHIFT ASSIGNMENTS AND ADVANCEMENT WITHIN THE DEPARTMENT

Any time a particular, regularly scheduled shift is vacated, all controllers who are interested in moving to that shift should be allowed to request reassignment to that shift. The requests should be made in writing to the communications supervisor or manager. Ideally, when there's competition for a shift assignment, a formal testing and interview process should take place; this is the fairest approach to filling any vacancy.

Because of the critical nature of the medical communicator's position, shift assignments in communications should never be made based solely on seniority. Although seniority should certainly be a consideration, many other factors must also be weighed. Among those factors are strengths and weaknesses of the personnel concerned, competency levels, time and schedule demands of the controllers' families, school schedules, overall knowledge of the system, cooperation, and the results of performance appraisals. The final decisions regarding shift reassignments and advancement into newly created or recognized positions should rest with the department manager.

## MAKING CRITICAL DECISIONS

There will be times when circumstances will place you in a position where you must make a time-critical procedural decision, and there are no specific policies or procedures in place to help you make that decision. Under these circumstances, it may help to apply this quick four-part test:

If you take the action you are considering, how will you feel:

Explaining what you have done to your boss
Explaining what you have done to the patient or the patient's family
Explaining what you have done to the media
Explaining what you have done while sitting on the witness stand in a courtroom

When these situations occur, stay calm and follow the general, obvious intent of policies that do exist, use your common sense, and always take whatever action will ensure the highest quality patient care. Whenever you are in doubt, you should have the opportunity to consult a manager or administrator for guidance and direction.

## SUMMARY AND REVIEW

1. What are some of the ways you can set yourself and your department up to win?

2. Where is your communications center located? Did the dis-

patchers themselves have any input into the design of the center?

3. What things should you and other communicators consider when designing your work area?

4. List the personality types of dispatchers in your system. How many can you identify?

5. How are shifts scheduled for your communicators? Are you consciously attempting to match supply with demand?

6. Can the actions that you routinely take in the communications center pass the four-part test for critical decisionmaking?

7. Why is medical certification important for medical dispatchers? Can certification as a medical dispatcher fill the same role in your system?

# Chapter 4

# SYSTEM STATUS MANAGEMENT

*"All I know is what I read in the papers."*
— Will Rogers

*"If you stop and think about it, you'll realize that three out of four persons do not know exactly what they're doing a large part of the time."*
— Gelett Burgess

WHAT IS IT, ANYWAY?

Many of the most progressive and highly productive EMS systems in this country utilize the combination of principles and practices known collectively as *System Status Management*. This approach to effectively meeting the demands on an EMS service was originated in the early 1970's by Jack Stout, who is today a nationally known EMS consultant. While you may hear many complicated definitions of system status management, it is, quite simply, *making the most efficient use of whatever resources are available at any given time, and planning effectively so that the resources available will be adequate to meet the demands made on your system.* System status management allows the manipulation and management of the status of the system to produce the best possible results. By Stout's own definition, it is "the art and science of matching the production capacity of an Emergency Medical Services system to the changing patterns of demand placed upon that system. It includes the formal or informal systems, protocols, and procedures which determine where the remaining ambulances will be when the next call comes in. More than that, SSM includes an overall fine-tuning of every aspect of operations to squeeze optimum productivity out of every unit hour produced."[1]

---

[1] See "Advanced SSM Workshop Selftest," The Fourth Party, Inc., 1987.

## GOALS OF SYSTEM STATUS MANAGEMENT

*"Results! Why, man, I have gotten a lot of results.
I know several thousand things that won't work."*
— *Thomas Alva Edison*

Why is it so important to the workers in any EMS system to function at all times in the most efficient way possible? There are many reasons and considerations. Among them is the realization that efficient system status management allows us to:

- Evenly distribute the work load among field crews
- Minimize emergency response times
- Staff to meet system work loads
- Properly maintain MICUs by allowing scheduled downtime for preventative maintenance
- Provide adequate coverage for all parts of our service area
- Reduce the stress of individual crew members by mixing emergency and nonemergency responses
- Preserve some 24-hour shifts by shifting some of the work load to short-shift crews
- Reduce the use of on-call crews
- Reduce nonemergency service delays
- Reduce mandatory overtime
- Develop schedules convenient to personnel (to allow for family time demands, school schedules, etc.)
- Develop a new experience base, both to guard the existing market and to bid for new markets
- Provide excellent customer service
- Contribute to the financial health of our service and our system

## OFF TO A ROCKY START: WHAT HAPPENED HERE?

*"If you don't lose your mind over
certain things, you haven't got a mind to lose."*
— *Johann Nestroy*

When the principles of system status management were first introduced, their value in emergency medical service was recognized quickly throughout the industry. Articles were published in trade journals and magazines, and organizations nationally known for their reputations for excellence began to put the principles into practice.

The more professional press the ideas received, the more systems began to implement their use. Administrators immediately recognized the soundness of the basic concepts, and, as is so typical of the personalities found in emergency medical service, system managers nationwide jumped into the process with both feet. Out of necessity, the original concepts were presented in general, theoretical terms.

Unfortunately, these general hypotheses were implemented *exactly and literally* in some service areas.

The result was predictable. With the misuse and mismanagement of SSM in systems across the country, the employees of the systems rebelled. When a response system is configured to function with a unit hour utilization ratio that is too high, the employees (both in the field and in communications) quickly burn out. If the deployment plan is too precise and too complicated, it actually generates more work for the employees, instead of less. When used improperly, the principles of system status management can be disastrous to morale.

Some system administrators stuck with it, worked through the process, and came up with workable, efficient system status plans. Others became discouraged and gave up. When you discuss system status management with members of different response systems, you will invariably hear opinions ranging from one extreme to the other. Negative views of the process are usually heard from those systems where SSM was attempted, and the attempt failed.

I have been employed in services where system status planning worked and in those where it did not, and I can tell you this: *The principles are sound, and when managed properly, they can greatly improve your overall system performance.* If you are a communicator in a service that has tried to use system status management and failed, do some current research on the subject, and then try it again.

## LEARNING FROM THE EXPERIENCE OF OTHERS: ALTHOUGH WE ARE SPECIAL, WE'RE NOT THAT DIFFERENT

Emergency medical service, as an industry, is still very young. For years, the assumption was almost universally held that EMS differed in basic ways from other types of enterprise. With careful study and documentation, we have finally learned that, in comparing our industry with others, there are more fundamental similarities than differences.

In any industry, specific methods of accomplishing that industry's goals are tried and proven over a period of time. Each time a new method or approach is tested, the principals in the related industry gain knowledge and add to their experience base. Gradually, the innovators in any industry learn that some things work better than others. Ideally, when the next new approach is introduced, it will be a logical improvement over the last successful method. Only in recent years have we in EMS finally learned that, in our pursuit of excellence, *it is not necessary to continually re-invent the wheel each time we attempt to improve.* Although adjustments and customization must certainly be performed to compensate for differences in the makeup of each service area, the principles used successfully in other parts of the country will generally also produce positive results in your service area.

Basic human nature leads us to believe that we, in our company or our service area, have demands, needs, and qualifying factors that are genuinely unique. When we can control our egos and make ourselves receptive to new ideas, we find that *types* of systems and *characteristics* of service areas generally fall into categories, and our unique needs are not at all uncommon.

## CHOOSING SMART OVER STUPID

*"When you have a choice to make and don't make it, that is in itself a choice."*
— *William James*

With the publication of the Eisenberg and Cayten studies[2], it was finally firmly established that response times and preplanned clinical treatment algorithms clearly impact the terminal prognoses for critical patients. The acknowledgment of the importance of clinical treatment algorithms led to the establishment of groups of physician medical advisors and rigorous quality assurance programs that rapidly became the goal for a national standard. Once the medical importance of response times had been recognized, the work to find ways to shorten those response times was begun in earnest. The refinement of system status management into "an art and a science" was the inevitable result of that effort.

Every EMS service in existence uses some type of system status management, whether or not it is recognized as such. The abundance of opinion, theory (both tested and untested), and actual detailed case studies of systems utilizing SSM now available in print will rapidly educate anyone who takes the time to read the information. Now that system status management has become part of the national standard for EMS services of even moderate size and call volume, it becomes the responsibility of all system administrators and policy makers to make choices; *it becomes their responsibility to make smart choices instead of stupid ones.*

Even a system that keeps ten units on the street at all times, utilizes all 24-hour shifts, and doesn't add more units to the staffing plan when call volume is high is using system status management. *That system's decision makers have made the choice not to provide flexibility in their system.*

Here's another example: At 2:00 in the morning, a system has eight crews asleep in 24-hour stations; then, all units except that on the far west side of the service area are dispatched on calls. If established procedure dictates that the one available crew will be left to sleep undisturbed, that, too, is a form of system status management. Whether directly or indirectly, whether consciously or without deliberate intent, the policy makers for that system have made a series of

---

[2] Stout, J.L.: "System Status Management: The Strategy of Ambulance Placement." Journal of Emergency Medical Services, 9 (5): 1983.

choices that will virtually guarantee a 20-minute response time for the critical patient in the eastern part of that service area at that hour of the morning.

Whether or not the deliberate, considered intent to harm the patient existed (and, as EMS professionals, we can safely assume it did not), the fact is that the patient will suffer. *This was a stupid choice.* Our goal must always be to make our systems as efficient and as responsive to our patients' needs as possible, through the use of *careful planning, extensive study, and consistently choosing smart over stupid.*

As a general rule, we should all try to live according to this guideline: *Don't act stupid in public.*

## MAKING INTELLIGENT DECISIONS

In what *initially seems* to be a direct contrast to the humanistic elements involved in providing high-quality patient care, modern emergency medical systems rely on numbers to function. In order to make smart choices, we must have reliable, usable information. *A smart choice is always based on the existence of data, not the lack of it.* The practical way to capture and store information relating to our profession is through the use of numbers.

If you are just beginning this process, you will wish to capture first the most basic numbers available. *Basic* can be defined in two different ways: the smallest size or quantity of information that is practical, and the types of information most important to our business. We must be able to identify the elements of what, when, where, and how much as they impact our system, and we must be able to identify them now. It is infinitely easier to capture information about an event as it occurs than it is to go back and try to recreate the event.

Information gathered after the fact is almost invariably unreliable. As soon as a moment has passed, our brains begin the process of distorting the memory of that moment. Again, this is a normal occurrence; it's the way our brains work.

If you ask any group of medical dispatchers which day of the week is busiest, they will *always* name a day that they work. One communications shift may tell you that Saturday afternoons are a living hell in the dispatch center, because call volume is incredibly high. When you look at the call volume demand, you see that Saturdays are no different than Fridays or Mondays; it is the communicators' *perceptions* of Saturdays that are different. When you have the opportunity to choose between hard statistical data and "feelings" or "hunches," always go with the hard data. There is a specific word for the mental processes that are called hunches because they are considered unusual; they are by definition unreliable. When you see consistent differences between the way field personnel and communicators perceive an event or a time period and the way the numbers look on paper, you should look not necessarily at changing the structure of the event, but at other factors that affect the employees' comfort levels during a designated time period.

What kind of numbers do we need? We need to know the total number of ambulances we have that we can put on the street. We need to know how many calls we run, during precisely measured time periods. We must know where the calls are. We must know the time periods in which the calls are run. We must know how long it takes to complete a transport. A listing of necessary information and suggested methods to record information about individual responses can be found in Chapter 15 of this text. Each of these pieces of information can be studied and used to improve system performance.

Sometimes, the key to effectively using information is based on simple logic. For example, if you are studiously analyzing historical data in a timely manner and adjusting staffing to meet your call demand, and your system is *still* not meeting response time requirements, where is one of the first places you should look for the opportunity to improve? The success of any system's performance relies on every member of the team conforming with certain standards, whether or not they know what those standards are. For each response mode category used in your system, calculate the elapsed time between when each call was received and when the assigned unit cleared from the call. If the average total elapsed task time for any category is greater than 60 minutes, that is where at least part of your problem lies. In the management of a large fleet where planning is measured in hourly increments, time overages in 5-minute increments quickly add up to time in hours. This is not secret information or a magic formula: it's simple common sense.

To provide yourself and your system with the information you need to work most effectively, there are common phrases and principles you will need to know.

## DEFINITIONS OF COMMON TERMS

A *unit hour* is one ambulance, fully equipped, fully staffed, and fully available for any use the system requires, for the time period of one hour.

*Unit hour demand* or *call volume* is the number of responses or transports (depending on what you're using the information for) during one hour of one particular day over a given period of time.

*Simple average demand* is the average (arithmetic mean) number of responses or transports occurring during any specific hour on a specific day of the week over a defined period of time. A time period of 20 weeks is suggested as the minimum with which to evaluate system demands. Evaluating the simple average demand for the two o'clock hour on Tuesday during a 20-week period, you will average 20 Tuesdays, or 20 two o'clock hours (see Figure 4.1).

*High average* demand, like the simple average, is calculated as an arithmetic mean. For effective planning, we must be able to predict not only *what* will happen (how many calls we will run), but *when*

50  *System Status Management*  Chap. 4

DAY: TUESDAY    HOUR: 0200    TIME PERIOD: JAN 1–MAY 22

| Date | Responses Made | Date | Responses Made |
|---|---|---|---|
| Jan. 6 | 13 | Mar. 17 | 16 |
| 13 | 15 | 24 | 22 |
| 20 | 12 | 31 | 17 |
| 27 | 17 | Apr. 7 | 15 |
| Feb. 3 | 15 | 14 | 13 |
| 10 | 16 | 21 | 16 |
| 17 | 21 | 28 | 17 |
| 24 | 14 | May 5 | 17 |
| Mar. 3 | 17 | 12 | 14 |
| 10 | 13 | 19 | 15 |

Figure 4.1 *Analysis of Call Volume. The simple average is the total number of responses divided by the number of weeks in the time period.* 315 divided by 20 = 15.75. *To calculate the high average, divide the response numbers into groups of four. Add the single highest numbers in each set of four, then divide by the number of sets.* High average = 17 + 21 + 22 + 17 + 17 = 94. 94 divided by 5 = 18.80. Peak average *is the sum of the highest numbers in two 10-week sets;* 21 + 22 = 43. 43 divided by 2 = 21.5. *The high actual is the highest single number occurring in the entire set of numbers.* High actual = 22.

(when we will run them). The high average provides more specific information than a simple average. To calculate the high average, first divide the response numbers for the reporting period into groups of four. Then identify the highest number in each set of four. Add these together and divide by the number of groups. This is the high average. This demand level can be expected to occur about once every month. If your system is prepared to handle this load, you will probably meet your response time requirements with about 75 percent reliability.[3]

*Peak average* is calculated as above, with another change in structure. Divide the complete group of numbers into smaller sets of ten. Identify the highest number in each group of ten. Now add these numbers together and average them. The peak average can be expected to occur about once every 10 weeks. If your system is prepared to handle this call volume load, you'll probably meet your response time requirements with about 90 percent reliability.[4]

The *high actual* call demand is the single highest number of responses ever occurring in the reporting period. If you could accurately calculate the high actual call demand, accurately predict the percentage of increase in call volume (due to increasing population, etc.), and consistently staff to meet or surpass these demands, you could theoretically meet your response time requirements 100 percent of the time.

*Peak-load staffing* is the logical practice of scheduling more avail-

---

[3] Advanced System Status Management Training Seminar, The Fourth Party, Inc., Copyright 1987.

[4] Ibid.

able unit hours when the unit hour demand is highest.

*Variable staffing* is the practice of combining shifts of several different types and lengths (8, 9, 10, 12, 24 hours, etc.) to provide the number of unit hours needed at any given time.

*Unit deployment* is the practice of strategically positioning available units as close as possible to the locations where the next calls will come in.

## USING THE RESULTS OF CALL DEMAND ANALYSES

To analyze information, you must establish a standardized format to help you do so. A simple Unit Hour Demand Analysis Worksheet is illustrated in Figure 4.2. Select any 20-week period in your system's past and review the data from all the different angles described earlier. Decide which standard of response time reliability (high average or peak average) your system should attempt, calculate the averages, and list them according to your system's standard on the unit hour demand analysis sheet. If your system provides both types of service, responses should be identified as emergency or nonemergency. Arrival times for nonemergency responses are frequently negotiable in times of system overload; emergency arrival times are not.

When you have the figures neatly organized and neatly noted on your neat little forms, *what do they mean?* These figures are not good or bad; they are neither right nor wrong. Comparing them with figures from other systems will not necessarily tell you anything at all. They must be reviewed and evaluated in terms of their relationships with other events, other happenings, and other sets of figures. Think relative.

One practical way to examine call demand analysis results, and to assign a value to them, is to *compare demand and supply*. In Figure 4.3 you will see a relationship defined between the unit hours staffed (supply) and the total call volume (unit hour demand). Each shift is identified, with its working hours listed. Total staffed unit hours for the day and time specified are totaled at the end of the report. The high average demand is subtracted from the unit hours staffed to provide the variance. In the system for which this specific report was prepared, any variance of 3 or less indicates the possibility of compromising patient care through extended response times (the service area is geographically very large and elongated on a north south axis); any variance of greater than 8 indicates the possibility that system productivity will be decreased, thus decreasing the financial profitability of the operation.

## LOST AND ADDED UNIT HOURS

It is also important in system status planning to recognize the practical difference between the number of unit hours *scheduled* and those

| UNIT HOUR DEMAND ANALYSIS ||||||||||||||||||||||||
|---|---|---|---|---|---|---|---|---|---|---|---|---|---|---|---|---|---|---|---|---|---|---|---|
| | Sunday ||| Monday ||| Tuesday ||| Wednesday ||| Thursday ||| Friday ||| Saturday ||| Totals |||
| Hour | E | N | T | E | N | T | E | N | T | E | N | T | E | N | T | E | N | T | E | N | T | E | N | T |
| 0000-0059 | 4 | 0 | 4 | 5 | 1 | 6 | 2 | 0 | 2 | 3 | 2 | 5 | 2 | 0 | 2 | 5 | 0 | 5 | 6 | 1 | 7 | 27 | 4 | 31 |
| 0100-0159 | 7 | 2 | 9 | 4 | 2 | 6 | 2 | 2 | 4 | 2 | 3 | 5 | 4 | 2 | 6 | 3 | 1 | 4 | 8 | 0 | 8 | 30 | 12 | 42 |
| 0200-0259 | 6 | 1 | 7 | 1 | 1 | 2 | 2 | 2 | 4 | 3 | 2 | 5 | 3 | 1 | 4 | 4 | 1 | 5 | 6 | 1 | 7 | 25 | 9 | 34 |
| 0300-0359 | 3 | 0 | 3 | 3 | 1 | 4 | 2 | 0 | 2 | 3 | 1 | 4 | 2 | 0 | 2 | 4 | 0 | 4 | 4 | 0 | 4 | 21 | 2 | 23 |
| 0400-0459 | 5 | 0 | 5 | 6 | 3 | 9 | 5 | 1 | 6 | 4 | 1 | 5 | 5 | 0 | 5 | 6 | 3 | 9 | 6 | 1 | 7 | 37 | 9 | 46 |
| 0500-0559 | 7 | 1 | 8 | 7 | 3 | 10 | 6 | 2 | 8 | 5 | 2 | 7 | 6 | 3 | 9 | 5 | 2 | 7 | 8 | 2 | 10 | 44 | 15 | 59 |
| 0600-0659 | 5 | 1 | 6 | 8 | 4 | 12 | 6 | 1 | 7 | 6 | 1 | 7 | 8 | 3 | 11 | 8 | 2 | 10 | 8 | 0 | 8 | 49 | 12 | 61 |
| 0700-0759 | 6 | 2 | 8 | 8 | 4 | 12 | 7 | 4 | 11 | 5 | 2 | 7 | 6 | 3 | 9 | 8 | 2 | 10 | 8 | 1 | 9 | 48 | 18 | 66 |
| 0800-0859 | 7 | 2 | 9 | 8 | 5 | 13 | 8 | 5 | 13 | 6 | 4 | 10 | 7 | 4 | 11 | 9 | 5 | 14 | 8 | 1 | 9 | 53 | 26 | 79 |
| 0900-0959 | 7 | 0 | 7 | 9 | 6 | 15 | 8 | 4 | 12 | 6 | 3 | 9 | 7 | 4 | 11 | 9 | 6 | 15 | 9 | 0 | 9 | 55 | 23 | 78 |
| 1000-1059 | 7 | 1 | 8 | 9 | 4 | 13 | 9 | 3 | 12 | 6 | 2 | 8 | 8 | 2 | 10 | 9 | 3 | 12 | 8 | 1 | 9 | 56 | 16 | 72 |
| 1100-1159 | 6 | 0 | 6 | 8 | 2 | 10 | 8 | 3 | 11 | 6 | 1 | 7 | 8 | 0 | 8 | 8 | 1 | 9 | 9 | 0 | 9 | 53 | 7 | 60 |
| 1200-1259 | 7 | 1 | 8 | 9 | 4 | 13 | 9 | 3 | 12 | 5 | 3 | 8 | 9 | 4 | 13 | 9 | 5 | 14 | 8 | 0 | 8 | 56 | 20 | 76 |
| 1300-1359 | 5 | 0 | 5 | 8 | 2 | 10 | 8 | 2 | 10 | 5 | 1 | 6 | 7 | 2 | 9 | 8 | 3 | 11 | 8 | 1 | 9 | 49 | 11 | 60 |
| 1400-1459 | 5 | 0 | 5 | 7 | 3 | 10 | 6 | 2 | 8 | 5 | 2 | 7 | 6 | 2 | 8 | 7 | 0 | 7 | 7 | 0 | 7 | 43 | 9 | 52 |
| 1500-1559 | 6 | 1 | 7 | 6 | 1 | 7 | 5 | 1 | 6 | 5 | 1 | 6 | 5 | 2 | 7 | 6 | 1 | 7 | 6 | 1 | 7 | 39 | 8 | 47 |
| 1600-1659 | 7 | 0 | 7 | 7 | 1 | 8 | 7 | 0 | 7 | 8 | 0 | 8 | 7 | 1 | 8 | 8 | 2 | 10 | 7 | 0 | 7 | 51 | 4 | 55 |
| 1700-1759 | 7 | 0 | 7 | 8 | 1 | 9 | 8 | 1 | 9 | 9 | 2 | 11 | 9 | 1 | 10 | 9 | 2 | 11 | 9 | 1 | 10 | 59 | 8 | 67 |
| 1800-1859 | 7 | 1 | 8 | 8 | 0 | 8 | 9 | 0 | 9 | 9 | 1 | 10 | 9 | 0 | 9 | 9 | 1 | 10 | 10 | 0 | 10 | 61 | 3 | 64 |
| 1900-1959 | 7 | 0 | 7 | 7 | 1 | 8 | 7 | 1 | 8 | 8 | 0 | 8 | 9 | 0 | 9 | 8 | 1 | 9 | 9 | 0 | 9 | 55 | 3 | 58 |
| 2000-2059 | 8 | 0 | 8 | 8 | 1 | 9 | 9 | 0 | 9 | 9 | 1 | 10 | 9 | 0 | 9 | 9 | 0 | 9 | 9 | 1 | 10 | 61 | 3 | 64 |
| 2100-2159 | 7 | 0 | 7 | 7 | 0 | 7 | 8 | 0 | 8 | 9 | 0 | 9 | 8 | 1 | 9 | 8 | 1 | 9 | 9 | 0 | 9 | 56 | 2 | 58 |
| 2200-2259 | 8 | 0 | 8 | 8 | 1 | 9 | 9 | 0 | 9 | 8 | 0 | 8 | 9 | 0 | 9 | 7 | 0 | 7 | 8 | 1 | 9 | 57 | 2 | 59 |
| 2300-2359 | 7 | 0 | 7 | 9 | 0 | 9 | 8 | 1 | 9 | 7 | 0 | 7 | 8 | 0 | 8 | 7 | 0 | 7 | 9 | 0 | 9 | 55 | 1 | 56 |
| Totals | 151 | 13 | 164 | 168 | 51 | 219 | 158 | 38 | 196 | 142 | 35 | 177 | 161 | 35 | 196 | 173 | 42 | 215 | 187 | 13 | 200 | 1140 | 227 | 1367 |

Figure 4.2  *Unit hour demand analysis worksheet*

Chap. 4  System Status Management

| Shift Type | 0 | 1 | 2 | 3 | 4 | 5 | 6 | 7 | 8 | 9 | 10 | 11 | 12 | 13 | 14 | 15 | 16 | 17 | 18 | 19 | 20 | 21 | 22 | 23 | Ttl |
|---|---|---|---|---|---|---|---|---|---|---|---|---|---|---|---|---|---|---|---|---|---|---|---|---|---|
| 09A | | | | | | | | | | | | | | | | | | | | | | | | | 0 |
| 09B | | | | | | | | | | | | | | | | | | | | | | | | | 0 |
| 09C | | | | | | | | | | | | | | | | | | | | | | | | | 0 |
| 09D | 1 | 1 | 1 | | | | | | | | | | | | | 1 | 1 | 1 | 1 | 1 | 1 | 1 | 1 | 1 | 12 |
| 09E | 1 | | | | | | | | | | | | | | | | | | | | | | | | 1 |
| 09F | | | | | | | | | | | | | | | | | | | | | | | | | 0 |
| 09G | 1 | 1 | | | | | | | | | | | | | | | | | | | | | | | 2 |
| 09H | | | | | | | | | | | | | | | | | | | | | | | | | 0 |
| 09I | | | | | | | | 1 | 1 | 1 | 1 | 1 | 1 | 1 | 1 | 1 | | | | | | | | | 9 |
| 09J | | | | | | | | | | | | | | | | | | | | | | | | | 0 |
| 09K | | | | | | | | | | | | | | | | | | | | | | | | | 0 |
| 09L | | | | | | | 1 | 1 | 1 | 1 | 1 | 1 | 1 | 1 | 1 | | | | | | | | | | 9 |
| 09M | | | | | | | | | | 1 | 1 | 1 | 1 | 1 | 1 | 1 | 1 | 1 | | | | | | | 9 |
| 09N | | | | | | | | | | | | | | | | | | | | | | | | | 0 |
| 09O | | | | | | | | | | 1 | 1 | 1 | 1 | 1 | 1 | 1 | 1 | 1 | | | | | | | 9 |
| 09P | | | | | | | | | 1 | 1 | 1 | 1 | 1 | 1 | 1 | 1 | 1 | | | | | | | | 9 |
| 09Q | | | | | | | | | | | | | | | | | | 1 | 1 | 1 | 1 | 1 | 1 | 1 | 7 |
| 09R | | | | | | | | | | | | | | | | | | | | | | | | | 0 |
| 09S | | | | | | | | | | | | | | | | | | | | | | | | | 0 |
| 09T | | | | | | | | 1 | 1 | 1 | 1 | 1 | 1 | 1 | 1 | 1 | | | | | | | | | 9 |
| 09U | | | | | | | | | | | | | | | | | | | | | | | | | 0 |
| 09V | | | | | | | | | 1 | 1 | 1 | 1 | 1 | 1 | 1 | 1 | 1 | | | | | | | | 9 |
| 09W | | | | | | | | | | | | | | | | | | | | | | | | | 0 |
| 09X | | | | | | | | | | | | | | | | | | | | | | | | | 0 |
| 09Y | 1 | 1 | | | | | | | | | | | | | | | | 1 | 1 | 1 | 1 | 1 | 1 | 1 | 9 |
| 09Z | 1 | | | | | | | | | | | | | | | | 1 | 1 | 1 | 1 | 1 | 1 | 1 | 1 | 9 |
| 12A | 1 | 1 | 1 | 1 | 1 | 1 | | | | | | | | | | | | | 1 | 1 | 1 | 1 | 1 | 1 | 12 |
| 12B | 1 | 1 | 1 | 1 | 1 | 1 | 1 | 1 | | | | | | | | | | | | | 1 | 1 | 1 | 1 | 12 |
| 12C | | | | | | | | | | | | | | | | | | | | | | | | | 0 |
| 12D | 1 | 1 | 1 | 1 | 1 | | | | | | | | | | | | | 1 | 1 | 1 | 1 | 1 | 1 | 1 | 12 |
| 12E | 1 | 1 | 1 | 1 | 1 | 1 | | | | | | | | | | | | | 1 | 1 | 1 | 1 | 1 | 1 | 12 |
| 12F | 1 | 1 | 1 | 1 | 1 | 1 | 1 | 1 | | | | | | | | | | | | | 1 | 1 | 1 | 1 | 12 |
| 12G | | | | | | | | | | | | | | | | | | | | | | | | | 0 |
| 12H | 1 | 1 | 1 | 1 | 1 | 1 | 1 | 1 | | | | | | | | | | | | | 1 | 1 | 1 | 1 | 12 |
| 12I | | | | | | | | | | | | | | | | | | | | | | | | | 0 |
| 12J | | | | | | | | | | | | | | | | | | | | | | | | | 0 |
| 12K | | | | | | | | | | | | | | | | | | | | | | | | | 0 |
| 12L | | | | | | | | | | | | | | | | | | | | | | | | | 0 |
| 12M | | | | | 1 | 1 | 1 | 1 | 1 | 1 | 1 | 1 | 1 | 1 | 1 | 1 | | | | | | | | | 12 |
| 12N | | | | 1 | 1 | 1 | 1 | 1 | 1 | 1 | 1 | 1 | 1 | 1 | 1 | | | | | | | | | | 12 |
| 12O | | | | | | | | | | | | | | | | | | | | | | | | | 0 |
| 12P | | | | | | | | | | | | | | | | | | | | | | | | | 0 |
| 12Q | 1 | 1 | | | | | | | | | | | | | | | 1 | 1 | 1 | 1 | 1 | 1 | 1 | 1 | 12 |
| 24A | 1 | 1 | 1 | 1 | 1 | 1 | 1 | | | | | | | | | | | | | | | | | | 7 |
| 24B | | | | | | | 1 | 1 | 1 | 1 | 1 | 1 | 1 | 1 | 1 | 1 | 1 | 1 | 1 | 1 | 1 | 1 | 1 | 1 | 17 |
| 24C | 1 | 1 | 1 | 1 | 1 | 1 | 1 | | | | | | | | | | | | | | | | | | 7 |
| 24D | | | | | | | | 1 | 1 | 1 | 1 | 1 | 1 | 1 | 1 | 1 | 1 | 1 | 1 | 1 | 1 | 1 | 1 | 1 | 17 |
| Staffed | 14 | 12 | 9 | 9 | 10 | 10 | 10 | 11 | 9 | 11 | 11 | 11 | 11 | 11 | 11 | 9 | 8 | 10 | 10 | 10 | 13 | 13 | 13 | 13 | 259 |
| EM Demand | 12 | 10 | 4 | 7 | 6 | 5 | 4 | 5 | 4 | 4 | 4 | 6 | 6 | 5 | 5 | 6 | 6 | 6 | 5 | 5 | 7 | 8 | 9 | 10 | 149 |
| NE Demand | 2 | 1 | 3 | 3 | 3 | 4 | 4 | 5 | 5 | 4 | 5 | 4 | 5 | 5 | 5 | 3 | 3 | 2 | 3 | 4 | 4 | 2 | 2 | 1 | 82 |
| Variance | 0 | 1 | 2 | -1 | 1 | 1 | 2 | 1 | 0 | 3 | 2 | 1 | 0 | 1 | 1 | 0 | -1 | 2 | 2 | 1 | 2 | 3 | 2 | 2 | 28 |

Mean Hourly Variance = 1.2 Unit Hours

Figure 4.3  *Unit hours staffed vs. unit hour demand for Saturday, 20 weeks ending 05/22*

actually *produced*. If a field unit is unavailable to respond to the needs of the system because of unexpected downtime for maintenance, a faulty or slipshod resupply procedure, or a policy of providing completely protected meal times, that lost time must be accounted for (see Figure 4.4). The Lost/Added Unit Hours Report is one method of documenting differences between the number of unit hours scheduled and produced during any specific time period. In this case, the reporting period is 24 hours long, beginning at 0000 and ending at 2359 on a given calendar date. An ambulance with a flat tire is clocked out of service at 1430; when the tire has been replaced, the unit is clocked into service at 1500. This half-hour of maintenance time was not previously scheduled; it is recorded and a running total is kept of downtime due to unplanned maintenance. A field EMT becomes ill during his shift and two and one-half hours pass before a replacement can be found. This unexpected downtime is logged to personnel. A field crew makes a call that keeps them out 47 minutes past their designated shift end time; this time is added under the category "late call." A regularly scheduled unit is sent out of the system on a long-distance transport that takes 6 hours and 15 minutes to complete. Time is recorded in elapsed hours and minutes. At the end of the reporting period, the hours and minutes are totaled by category and converted into hours and hundredths of hours. The total change in time is then added to or subtracted from the unit hours scheduled to calculate the actual number of unit hours produced.

If you have never examined this aspect of your system's performance, you may be both amazed and appalled at the amount of time being lost in small increments. The simple recognition that the situation exists usually leads to simplifying and streamlining in-place procedures.

## RESPONSE TIME REPORTING

Response time is a phrase that may initially be misleading; it should not measure *only* the time elapsed while the field crew is actually driving to a specified address. The total response time for any run begins as soon as the call is officially received. When a CAD system is in use, this will be the time the call is entered. Where a manual dispatch system is employed, the "call received time" is the time at which the last of the three critical elements of data needed for dispatch (incident location, call-back number, and presumptive patient condition) is received by the call-taker. The response time ends when the field unit arrives at the scene of the incident.

Most prehospital care systems are required to comply with an established standard of response time performance. The elapsed total response time must be calculated (either by a CAD system or manually) in minutes and seconds for each call run. At the end of each reporting period (daily, monthly, quarterly, seasonally, and/or yearly), a system's *response time compliance* must be calculated.

Even in systems where performance is not required by a legally

Chap. 4     System Status Management

| LOST/ADDED UNIT HOURS REPORT | | | | DATE 01/01    DAY Monday | PAGE / OF / |
|---|---|---|---|---|---|
| Unit | Shift | In | Out | Reason | (+,−) Time |
| 7 | 9A | 1500 | 1430 | 6 - flat tire | −:30 |
| 21 | 12C | 1140 | 0910 | 9 - EMT ill | −2:30 |
| 33 | 9D | 1500 | 1547 | 12 - Emergency Call | +:47 |
| 42 | 12N | 1815 | 1200 | 11 | −6:15 |

| | |
|---|---|
| 1. Shift start late, unknown reason | 8. Resupply during shift |
| 2. Shift start late, vehicle repair | 9. Personnel problem during shift −2.50 |
| 3. Shift start late, equipment repair | 10. Placed unavailable by admin. |
| 4. Shift start late, personnel late | 11. Out of system: long dist. txp. −6.25 |
| 5. Shift start late, short supplies | 12. Shift held over: late call +.78 |
| 6. Vehicle repair during shift −.50 | 13. Shift held over: coverage |
| 7. Equip repair/replace during shift | 14. Other (detail): |
| Field supervisor on duty: Anderson | Comms. supervisor on duty: Jones |

Figure 4.4   *Lost/added unit hours report*

binding contract, response time compliance reports should be provided in a timely manner to the chief, commander, owners, department or section managers, and field or line workers in any system. Without a goal to work toward or a standard to measure by and compare with, not many of us will be motivated to improve our performance. And, even in areas where no contract or official time-critical responsibility exists, it is always wise to have response time performance information readily available for legal reasons.

How is response time compliance calculated? Take, for example, a system that prioritizes requests for ambulance service into five broad categories. A priority 1 response indicates a situation that is considered emergent and life-threatening. Priority 1 responses are made with lights and siren; first responders are also requested. The ambulance must arrive on the scene in less than 9 minutes (for practical purposes, this means within 8 minutes and 59 seconds). Priority 2 means emergent, but not life-threatening; the responding ambulance runs with lights and siren, but first responders are not dispatched. The response time requirement for priority 2 calls is less than 10 minutes. Priority 3 calls are not considered critical enough to make an emergency response, but not stable enough to be scheduled into the queue for a routine patient transport. The closest unit is sent, and is required to proceed immediately to the scene without delay. Lights and siren are not used. Response times should be less than 15 minutes. Priority 4 calls are routine patient transports scheduled 3 or more hours in advance. These take time precedence over uncomplicated Priority 5 requests, which are routine transports not scheduled ahead of time. The time clock for priority 4 and 5 responses is set at 1 hour. Any response time that does not meet the requirements for its prioritization category is called a *response time exception*. The reporting day changes at midnight with the change of the calendar date.

At the end of each reporting day, a count is made of the total number of transports made in each category, along with the number of response time exceptions for calls where patients were transported in each grouping. Dry runs or calls where no patient was transported are not included in compliance calculations. The number of exceptions is subtracted from the number of total transports. The number of "good" response times of each priority is divided by the total number of transports of that priority. The resulting number is the compliance percentage for that priority of response.

On an average day in the system just described, 135 priority 1 responses are made. Of those responses, 116 result in patients being transported to hospitals. On 8 calls, the response time is 9 minutes or longer; by subtracting, we find that 108 responses are within the time requirements for priority 1 calls. When we divide 116 by 108, we calculate that our units were "on time" for priority 1 calls 93.10 percent of the time during this reporting day.

Calculating response time compliance percentages gives an accurate picture of our performance; averaging response times does not. Cumulative totals are calculated throughout the month, to provide a month-end compliance figure for all categories. Quarterly, seasonal, and annual reports can be generated from these monthly statistics.

## TRACKING THE WILD EXCEPTION

*Every time* a unit generates a response time that does not meet your response time requirement criteria, careful and thorough documentation of the response must be completed. You can't fix a problem if you don't know it exists.

Every time your system generates an extended response time, you need to identify a number of bits of detailed information. The goal is to identify any factor or factors that may have caused this response time exception, and that can be prevented in the future. Is there one crew that has extended "chute" times? Is there a post or station that has poor freeway access during rush hours? Is there a specific day or hour when your system generates more response exceptions than in others? Is it time to revise your deployment plan?

Response time exception reporting may be accomplished by manual standardized forms (Figure 4.5) or by entering data into a simple calculating spreadsheet stored in a freestanding personal computer or CAD system. It is very helpful to generate response time exception reports which identify all of a selected group of factors monthly; by viewing the problem from a broader perspective, you will see patterns and trends develop. Then you can isolate and identify recurring problems, and correct them.

## UNIT DEPLOYMENT AND POST SELECTION

*Remember that in a crisis situation, a planned response is better than an unplanned response.* That's all a unit deployment plan is: a plan for where to position your available ambulances, so they will be close to the calls as they come in. Designing a unit placement plan and selecting posting locations is not something you can just run out and do; like every other aspect of this job, it requires careful and considered thought and planning.

### The Strategy of Ambulance Placement

The initial step in building your first plan for unit placement is to construct demand maps. This process can be as complex as writing a lengthy computer program, or as simple as sticking straight pins in a map.

If you're working manually, draw or trace a large, very simple line representation of your service area (see Figure 4.6). Identify a minimum number of pertinent landmarks (your system headquarters building, hospitals, fire stations, etc.). Make many, many copies of the map. Gather the data from the designated reporting period (again, a 20-week period is suggested for all your statistical computations, since

## RESPONSE TIME EXCEPTION REPORT

| Day Monday | Date 01/01 | Priority 1 | Type of Call 160 |
|---|---|---|---|
| Incident # 2195 | Encounter Address 3201 North Main | | |
| District 01 | Responded From P07 | Predicted Response Time 7.5 min | |
| Unit Number 27 | Field Crew Names/ID #s Davis/400; Adams/475 | | |
| System Level at Dispatch 8 | Supervisor on Duty Johnson | | Notified? N |
| Reason for Long Response Time Unit at Post 1 took emergency call at 1726; Medic 27 was moved up to Post 1 from Post 7 at 1727. This call came in at 1728. | | | |
| Radio Operator Brown/450 | Call-Taker Jones/465 | | Call-Taker Green/420 |
| Reviewed by J. Smith, System Status Manager | | | Date 01/02 J. Smith |

## RESPONSE TIME EXCEPTION REPORT

| Day Monday | Date 01/01 | Priority 1 | Type of Call 330 |
|---|---|---|---|
| Incident # 3204 | Encounter Address 1405 Maple Street | | |
| District 02 | Responded From P02 | Predicted Response Time 2.1 min | |
| Unit Number 7 | Field Crew Names/ID #s Hill/416; Jordan/421 | | |
| System Level at Dispatch 6 | Supervisor on Duty Johnson | | Notified? Y |
| Reason for Long Response Time Crew had long chute time (3:07) took improper routing and got caught in heavy traffic; when they attempted to reroute around the traffic, they got lost. | | | |
| Radio Operator Jones/465 | Call-Taker Brown/450 | | Call-Taker Green/420 |
| Reviewed by J. Smith, System Status Manager | | | Date 01/02 J. Smith |

Figure 4.5 *Response time exception report*

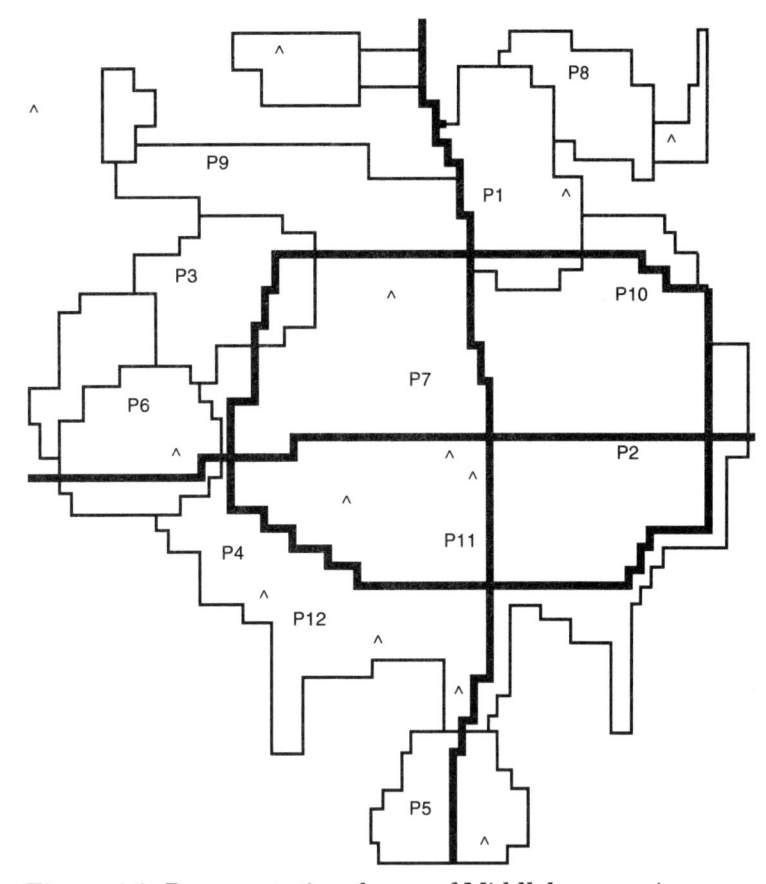

Figure 4.6 *Representational map of Middleburg service area*

it's the lowest number that can be divided by both 4 and 10). Using one map for each hour of each day (yes, that's 168 maps), mark the location from which each patient was transported. Use a different color or shape to mark transports that had long response times. At the end of the process, you will be able to identify the total number of transports and the long response times that occurred in each area (see Figure 4.7).

Making Your Post Selections

If life was simple, all you would have to do at this point is buy or lease quarters for your ambulance stations exactly where the highest concentrations of demand are marked on the maps. Unfortunately, there are many other elements to be considered in the strategy of unit placement, such as:

- *Financial concerns.* How much will it cost? In many areas, client cities or city governments will provide buildings for ambulance substations at reduced cost or no cost at all. (Yes, overall system profitability *is* your concern.)
- *Access.* Is there adequate access from the property location to major thoroughfares? What about to surrounding parts of the service area? Are nearby outlets congested during rush hour?

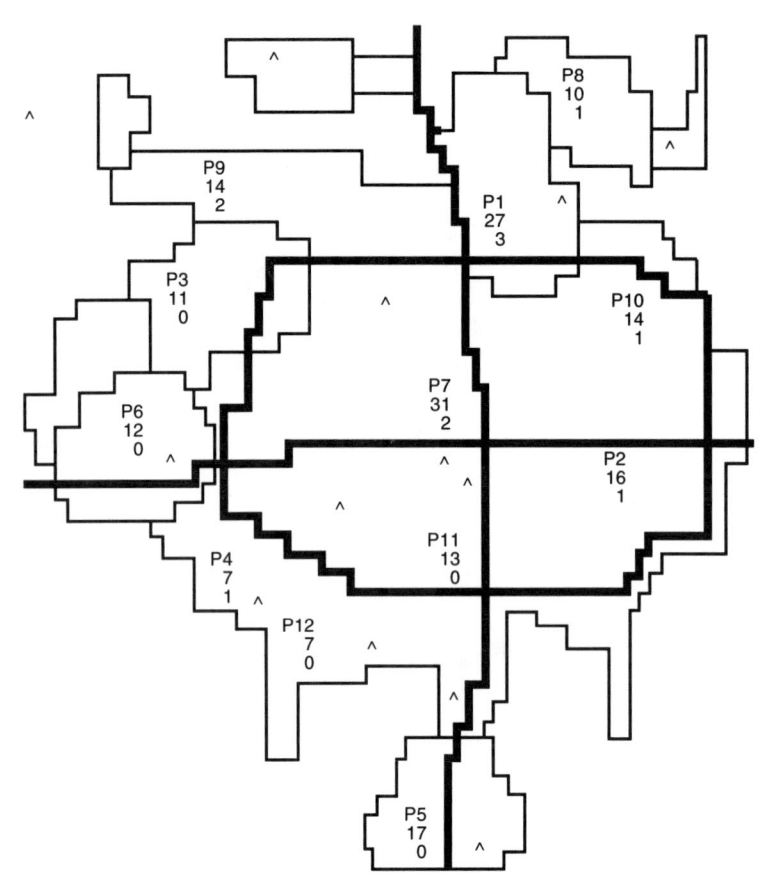

Figure 4.7 Middleburg service area response time problem map

- *Suitability.* Is this location an appropriate place for an ambulance substation? Can the ambulance be secured inside a garage or bay? Is the area safe and "respectable"? Will the presence of the station disturb those living in a residential neighborhood?
- *Geographic considerations.* By using strictly statistical demand criteria for placement, are you condemning the citizens of an isolated area to routinely long response times in life-threatening situations? If you literally "can't get there from here" in less than 10 minutes, look at your options again.
- *Street-corner posting.* While using a combination of some permanent "core" stations and some easily changeable street-corner posting locations is preferable, choose the second option with care. How many hours each day will crews be required to post in parking lots, etc.? Does the weather get very hot or very cold in your area? Could a crew be required to sit in their unit in subzero weather for several hours at a time? The issue of crew comfort must be thoroughly considered in this process.

When you have made logical location selections using all these criteria, identify each location with a number or a letter. Now you are ready to continue with the process of building a complete unit deployment plan.

### Consideration of System Levels

The *system level* is defined as the number of available units in the service area at a given time. A system with 12 available units is said to be at Level 12. It is very important, especially if your system uses 24-hour shifts, that you consider your predicted system levels as you confirm posting locations and designate the priority in which they are to be covered.

In combination with a number of 9- and 12-hour shifts, my system at one time still used three 24-hour stations to serve relatively remote, low-volume areas. Our team of system status planners (and I was one of them) once designed a beautiful, logical, very precise deployment plan which met both the statistical and geographic needs of our area. There was only one problem: *When we implemented the plan, the system level never got high enough for the 24-hour crews to return to their home stations.* They were either running calls or moving for coverage all day and all night. Their fatigue levels went through the roof. Very real concerns for crew safety and patient care led us to quickly revise the plan.

### Writing the Plan

Once you have familiarized your team with call volume demand, predictable system levels, and acceptable options for post locations, you can begin the process of actually writing the deployment plan. You may record the plan on maps, on a log form (see Figure 4.8), or both for easy reference.

Look at your demand map for the hour 0000–0059 on Sunday, Day 1. If you had only one available ambulance, where should you place it? Record the information, then move to system Level 2. If you had two available ambulances, where should you position them? Which post should you "cover" first? Record the information, and continue through the remaining days and hours.

### Implementing the New Deployment Plan

What should the finished deployment plan look like? This will vary with the needs of the individual service area. It should not only be as *simple,* but as *uncomplicated* (think about that) as possible. The first plan you put into practice will not be perfect; as you use it, you will discover areas where beneficial adjustments can be made. You will also find room for improvement in your second revised plan, and your third, and so on. The process is never over, since population concentrations and demand patterns constantly change.

When implementing your plan, remember these critical points:

- Don't look for the "right" plan; you will never find it. There is no permanent right answer. As demand patterns change in your service area, the plan must change with them.

Unit Deployment Plan for Sunday, Day 1, Hour 10

| | | | | | | | | | | | | | | | |
|---|---|---|---|---|---|---|---|---|---|---|---|---|---|---|---|
| 2 | | | | | | | | | | | | | | | |
| 2 | 6 | | | | | | | | | | | | | | |
| 2 | 6 | 3 | | | | | | | | | | | | | |
| 2 | 6 | 3 | 14 | | | | | | | | | | | | |
| 2 | 6 | 3 | 14 | 5 | | | | | | | | | | | |
| 2 | 6 | 3 | 14 | 5 | 21 | | | | | | | | | | |
| 2 | 6 | 3 | 14 | 5 | 21 | 20 | | | | | | | | | |
| 2 | 6 | 3 | 14 | 5 | 21 | 20 | 7 | | | | | | | | |
| 2 | 6 | 3 | 14 | 5 | 21 | 20 | 7 | 10 | | | | | | | |
| 2 | 6 | 3 | 14 | 5 | 21 | 20 | 7 | 10 | 8 | | | | | | |
| 2 | 6 | 3 | 14 | 5 | 21 | 20 | 7 | 10 | 8 | 1 | | | | | |
| 2 | 6 | 3 | 14 | 5 | 21 | 20 | 7 | 10 | 8 | 1 | 12 | | | | |
| 2 | 6 | 3 | 14 | 5 | 21 | 20 | 7 | 10 | 8 | 1 | 12 | 9 | | | |
| 2 | 6 | 3 | 14 | 5 | 21 | 20 | 7 | 10 | 8 | 1 | 12 | 9 | 13 | | |
| 2 | 6 | 3 | 14 | 5 | 21 | 20 | 7 | 10 | 8 | 1 | 12 | 9 | 13 | 4 | |
| 2 | 6 | 3 | 14 | 5 | 21 | 20 | 7 | 10 | 8 | 1 | 12 | 9 | 13 | 4 | 11 |
| 2 | 6 | 3 | 14 | 5 | 21 | 20 | 7 | 10 | 8 | 1 | 12 | 9 | 13 | 4 | 11 | 17 |
| 2 | 6 | 3 | 14 | 5 | 21 | 20 | 7 | 10 | 8 | 1 | 12 | 9 | 13 | 4 | 11 | 17 | 18 |

| Plan Number: 2A | Date In Effect: 06/01 | Date Plan Reviewed: 06/10 |
|---|---|---|
| Date Plan Reviewed: 09/10 | By: S. Smith | By: B. Adams |
| | | Date Plan Reviewed: 12/03 |
| | | By: S. Smith |

Figure 4.8 *Unit deployment plan*

- Don't try to make your plan too precise. Consider the frequency of post move-ups for field crews, and keep them to the absolute minimum that will provide response times that are acceptable from the standpoint of patient care.
- Don't implement a system status plan until you have provided education about system status management to personnel both in communications and the field.

## MEASURING PRODUCTIVITY

*Productivity* or *unit hour utilization* must be consistently evaluated and studied from two different angles to provide us with a broad perspective of how our system is performing. Productivity must be measured both to determine the amount of work being performed by the field crews and to discover what the financial status of the system will be in the future.

How is productivity measured? Although many intangible elements can be considered, this process can be reduced to the use of a simple mathematical formula. *The total number of transports divided by the number of unit hours produced equals the transport productivity index.*

On a given day in a hypothetical system, a total of 211 responses of all priorities were made. Of these, 153 resulted in patient transport. The number of unit hours scheduled was 404. Eleven hours and 45 minutes of available time were lost to maintenance, supply, training, and so on, resulting in 392.25 actual unit hours produced. Overall system *response productivity* is equal to 211 divided by 392.25, or 0.538. This indicates that field personnel actually worked just over half the hours they were on duty, *not counting post move-ups*. To calculate *transport productivity*, divide 153 by 392.25. The resulting figure is 0.390. This shows that field personnel were hypothetically generating revenue more than one third of their time on duty. Response and transport productivity, or unit hour utilization, can also be calculated by shift type. Logically, the amount of time spent making post move-ups should be factored into the response productivity equation, but should not be included in transport unit hour utilization.

As with most other aspects of system status management, there is no right or magic number for unit hour utilization. A variety of factors can and do influence the successful operation of any system; the *right* number is the one that strikes a balance in *your* system. Some systems can support a utilization ratio of .500; in other services, employees burn out at .400 or less. There is a number (at the high end of your possible scale) at which a for-profit system will produce revenue over and above expenses; at this point, your operation will show a financial gain. On the other hand, if unit hour utilization becomes too high, employee fatigue increases beyond an acceptable level. Very high utilization will also, at some point, make compliance with response time requirements difficult or impossible. Only time, experience, and careful analysis will establish the right balance for your system.

It is important for line medical dispatchers to understand the effect that each of their actions in the communications center has on the compliance and profitability of an emergency medical response system. In a system with rigid response time requirements, just one extended response time each day due to an inappropriate dispatch decision can knock the organization out of contractual compliance. If communicators do not conscientiously record lost unit hours, utilization cannot be computed accurately and profitability predictions can't be made correctly. It becomes impossible for administrators to precisely allocate resources for upcoming needs and successfully plan for the future. When planning is precise and an organization is financially successful, the employees realize visible, tangible benefits.

Again, each medical dispatcher must realize that every action produces a result; every action has a consequence. Work at seeing the "big picture." Watch your system's performance closely, and learn the possible effects (whether positive or negative) that each of your actions may have. Why? Because as an efficient, responsible medical communicator, you are capable of making positive contributions toward satisfactory response time performance and the financial well-being of your organization.

## SUMMARY AND REVIEW

1. What is system status management?

2. What are the goals of system status management?

3. What form of system status management is in use in your system? Are the choices you are making smart or stupid?

4. Make some telephone calls; write some letters. Contact medical communicators in other parts of the country. Ask what their service area is like. What are their guidelines regarding the use of system status management, telephone triage, pre-arrival instructions, and so on? Is there a national *norm*? How does your system differ from those in other areas? How is it the same?

5. Define the following terms: unit hour, unit hour demand, simple average demand, high average demand, peak average demand, peak-load staffing, variable staffing, and unit deployment.

6. What response mode categories are in use in your area? What are the response time requirements for each category?

7. Define unit hour utilization.

8. In a city- or county-supported EMS system, what are the advantages of simultaneously maintaining compliance with response time requirements and a high unit hour utilization ratio?

# Chapter 5

# ROLES AND RESPONSIBILITIES OF THE MEDICAL COMMUNICATOR

*"Work - work - work, till the brain begins to swim,
work - work - work, till the eyes are heavy and dim."*
— *Thomas Hood, "The Song of the Shirt"*

The medical communicator occupies a critical position within any emergency medical service system. She/he is the initial and primary contact point for persons needing medical assistance, and it is through the professional communicator that the citizen can be assisted in providing initial life-saving care to an injured or ill individual. In addition, the SSC provides a channel for communications among elements of the entire EMS system and between EMS providers and other public safety agencies. By carrying out these tasks effectively, the medical dispatcher can significantly contribute to a reduction in the frequency of death and the severity of residual disabilities resulting from accidents and illnesses. The dispatcher is responsible for providing information about special or hazardous scene situations to ensure the safety of responding personnel. She/he is responsible at all times for the status of the entire service area. These responsibilities must never be taken lightly; when you think about it, this can be a scary job. When you are comprehensively trained, properly supplied, and continually motivated to excel, it can also be more fun than any other work you've ever done.

## INITIAL CONTACT WITH THE PUBLIC

Always remember that as a medical communicator, you may provide the first and only exposure a citizen has to your emergency response system. What kind of impression will you leave with those who call for your help? Will you be helpful and supportive, or adversarial and antagonistic? If citizens and media reps with scanners listen to your voice on the radio, will they hear a competent professional or a terrified amateur? Calm and professional behavior is essential for a medical communicator; however, these qualities alone are not enough. In the dispatcher's role, you have to take that extra step. *You do whatever it takes to provide whatever assistance is needed by all who rely on you.*

## CHANNELING COMMUNICATIONS

One of your many tasks is to provide a vital communications link among different elements of the emergency response system. Picture yourself as a sophisticated conduit for all the little pieces of information that must move from one entity to another each day. The importance, suitability, and relevance of each bit of information must constantly be prioritized and reprioritized. The transfer of data should be quick and clean.

## CONCERN FOR CREW SAFETY

Among the pieces of information you will process each shift are indicators of conditions on the scene of all working medical incidents. You must consistently identify and relay those bits of data that may affect the safety of your field personnel on any scene. Some situations are clear and obvious from the outset; others may only provide clues to the circumstances that exist at any incident location. When the hazardous elements of a situation cannot be clearly and quickly identified, you have the obligation to pass information on to those responding, and to anticipate and prepare for their needs.

## POLICIES AND PROCEDURES

As a communicator, your responsibility is not only to be thoroughly familiar with stated or written policies for dispatch personnel and situations. You must also possess a current knowledge of field policies, procedures, and protocols. You must be able to participate in quality assurance programs for field personnel; how can you know if the progression of events during any response is satisfactory if you don't know the rules? You may also, at any time, be asked for advice or assistance in dealing with problems not frequently encountered by field personnel. You are a readily available resource for your field crews; expect to be asked to help in difficult or unusual circumstances.

## SYSTEM STATUS PLANNING AND ON-LINE MANAGEMENT

Every medical communicator should know the basic principles of system status management, even if the techniques are not consciously or deliberately being used in her/his system. Remember that every system uses some kind of system status management, whether the players are aware of it or not. In the newly defined dispatcher's role, the total responsibility for the efficient management of the emergency response system is yours.

## GEOGRAPHIC KNOWLEDGE

The medical dispatcher must have current and accurate knowledge of the geographic components of her/his service area. Your knowledge level should surpass even that of your field responders.

A thorough knowledge of your service area is first required to alert a specific crew even before the formal dispatch. With very few exceptions, you should know which unit is closest to a call as soon as you hear a street name or telephone number exchange. Pre-alerting units contributes to achieving the goal of providing your system's clients with the shortest possible response time.

When sufficient information to dispatch has been obtained, your geographic knowledge is tested again. In order to choose correctly when two or more units are close to being equidistant from an incident location, you must be aware of street access availability and traffic patterns.

While the response is active, you may be asked again to demonstrate your expert geographic knowledge. Even in heavily-populated urban areas where professional maps are available, pages can be lost or maps misplaced altogether. You must be ready at any time to provide supplemental routing instructions.

## KNOWLEDGE OF YOUR EQUIPMENT

Today's radio, telephone, and computer equipment is made up of millions and millions of tiny little parts; at one time or another, each one of those parts is guaranteed to malfunction. In addition, many field people will assume that, because you know how to talk on the radio, you also know how the radio works (silly, I know). Field personnel may even consult you when they develop problems with their mobile or portable radio equipment.

You should be familiar with basic trouble-shooting procedures for every piece of equipment in the communications center. Included in various systems are telephone lines, radio consoles, computers (both mainframes and smaller personal computers), printers, and the like. Even if you're not an electronics expert, you should at least be able to perform a series of basic, initial steps to repair equipment that malfunctions, while you wait for the real repair people to arrive. You should be familiar with emergency procedures in the communications center. What would you do if the power to your building was interrupted? If the incoming telephone lines went out? If your CAD system crashed?

You must also know where to call for technical support if your basic trouble-shooting efforts don't work. Who repairs your printers? Do the same people work on the telephones and the radio system? Are there emergency numbers to call when a problem occurs after hours? *The time to research this information and to practice troubleshooting techniques is before the equipment malfunctions.*

## HANDLING ROUTINE RADIO AND TELEPHONE TRAFFIC

As an everyday part of your job, you will be expected to effectively perform many tasks at once. You must competently handle radio and telephone traffic, even under extremely busy conditions. Each time a response is required, you must calmly and smoothly activate the emergency response system. You must methodically deal with situations that are crises in themselves. You are expected to perform efficiently and professionally even in times of communications center overload.

## RECEIVING AND PROCESSING CALL INFORMATION

Each time your dispatch center receives a call for help, you must follow a prescribed course of action. You must ask specific questions, and make rational decisions based on the answers to those questions. You must triage every call by telephone, always following your system's approved telephone protocols. You must provide comfort and reassurance to the caller, and instruct the caller in life-saving intervention techniques whenever practical. You must possess sufficient skill in remote communication to elicit every piece of information that will enable your system to provide the most suitable response possible.

## TELEPHONE TRIAGE AND REMOTE-DIRECTED INTERVENTION

Each medical dispatcher must develop and maintain basic and advanced telephone interviewing skills. Since these skills differ drastically from those practiced in direct communication, considerable study and practice are frequently necessary to become proficient in this area.

The communicator must also be highly skilled in various calming techniques, since the caller in an uncontrolled panic state is usually unable to provide the critical information needed to dispatch the emergency response.

## RESOURCE MANAGEMENT

Appropriate resource allocation is an art form that often goes unrecognized. The key to performing effective resource management is in preparation. You must know not only what assets your system can provide, but what human and mechanical resources are available from surrounding communities. You must develop expertise in working in the anticipatory mode, in order to be ready if your skills are called upon.

## RANGE OF SERVICES

One of the most frightening and irritating things that can happen to a citizen in any service area is to have what is perceived as a "simple question" left unanswered. When a dispatcher says, "I'm not sure, I'll need to check on that for you," the typical reaction from the caller is, "Why *don't* you know? You're *dispatching* there. I thought you were supposed to know everything."

Medical communicators are supposed to be "the answer people." Don't act stupid in public. *Know before the phone rings exactly what services your system does and does not provide, and why.*

## INTERFACING WITH OTHER DEPARTMENTS AND AGENCIES

Just as the dispatcher often provides the initial, and sometimes only, contact with the general public, she or he is often the system's only contact with other departments and agencies. Employees of hospitals, treatment centers, and neighboring police and fire departments often base their evaluation of your entire system solely on your telephone or radio attitude. Courteous, professional behavior is especially crucial when dealing with outside agencies.

## SYSTEM STATUS AND SYSTEM COMPLIANCE WITH OBLIGATIONS

As a medical dispatcher, you are responsible at all times for the overall response readiness of your system. It is your job to make sure each crew has what they need to efficiently function. You must make necessary post move-ups to ensure that all portions of your service area have the availability of a rapid emergency response. You should watch the time as your units are responding, and know when they are approaching the acceptable upward limit of time for any response. Since your actions and those of your co-workers are so intimately linked with the performance outcome for your system, I strongly recommend that statistical computations for response time compliance and productivity be conducted within the communications department itself. If you have a working knowledge of how your system's statistics are prepared, you will better understand how each of your actions impacts the system overall.

## QUALITY ASSURANCE

What better place to assist with systemwide quality control than in the dispatch center? You should already be monitoring response readiness and elapsed response times; in many systems, the professional communicators also hear patient reports and physician orders.

Monitoring and assessing the effectiveness of patient reports to hospitals, physician orders solicited or given, medical treatment administered, and choice of transport modes are an integral part of the medical communicator's job. Channels for automatic feedback to the system's clinical division should be clearly identified and agreed upon.

In addition, dispatchers must establish and maintain their own quality assurance programs. In this way, they can continually evaluate the effectiveness of themselves and their co-workers.

## WORKING AS A TEAM PLAYER

Although each individual communicator must identify and reach a high personal performance standard, each must also achieve a superlative skills level in participatory teamwork. The team approach produces superior results in almost every situation; this is especially true in emergency medical service.

Truly professional medical communicators do much more than merely walk through the mechanics of the dispatcher's job. They provide cooperation, encouragement, and support to all members of the response team: other communicators, field crews, first responders, field operations supervisors, and ancillary staff members from the public relations, supply, and maintenance departments. Only when all members of the team interact closely and professionally can an EMS system contribute to the best possible outcome in any situation.

## INSTANT REPLAY

That's a lot of stuff. To summarize, here is a condensed version of the medical communicator's roles, responsibilities, and job duties. The professional medical dispatcher must:

- Have a thorough working knowledge of policies and procedures in place in the system, and must consistently follow those policies and procedures
- Develop and utilize understanding of advanced principles of system status planning and on-line management
- Become familiar with the geographic components of both the service area and surrounding communities, and must provide specific routing instructions when needed
- Have a thorough working knowledge of the CAD system or other critical equipment, for example, dispatch consoles, paging system, telephones, and printers, and must be able to perform basic troubleshooting procedures for all
- Handle EMS message traffic in a prompt, accurate, courteous, and professional manner so as to assist callers for EMS assistance and EMS responders
- Obtain from each caller requesting medical assistance the necessary information to dispatch appropriate personnel and vehicles in the appropriate response mode
- Have the knowledge and capability to correctly utilize the medi-

cally approved dispatch prioritization protocols when medical assistance is requested. She/he must also have the knowledge and capability to correctly utilize the medically approved pre-arrival protocols when emergency medical assistance is needed by a caller until EMS personnel arrive at the incident location

- Acquire the necessary telephone skills in calming techniques to break the "hysteria threshold" and enable the SSC to give the caller necessary assistance
- Have the ability to recognize and recall the emergency medical services resources available in the service area, their capabilities and limitations, and their geographic locations and response areas
- Have a thorough knowledge of the range of services provided by the system
- Allocate EMS resources properly in response to emergency medical needs by application of appropriate decision making and medically approved and prioritized dispatch protocols
- Have a thorough knowledge of the ways in which the communications center interfaces with other departments in the system and with other agencies in and surrounding the service area
- Constantly monitor the status of the system and work to maintain system compliance with contract requirements
- Participate in the department's quality assurance and continuing education programs
- Work as a team member to provide a caring, supportive, professional environment for fellow medical dispatchers, callers, field crews, support services, administrative staff, ancillary medical professionals, and the citizens in the service area.

## ACTIVITIES INAPPROPRIATE TO THE MEDICAL COMMUNICATOR

The professional medical communicator *does not:*

- Fail to follow the system status plan
- Tell EMS personnel what to do, but *does* channel information and establish the necessary communications links to enable EMS personnel to carry out their responsibilities
- Diagnose the medical problems of a patient, but *does* provide the information necessary to institute life-saving emergency care in response to signs and symptoms reported by a caller
- Second-guess EMS personnel on the scene and try to make long-distance patient care determinations
- Give preferential treatment to certain personnel at the expense of others
- React with hostility to hostile callers or make judgment decisions based on a caller's demeanor or attitude
- Allow past experiences with callers to adversely influence dispatch decisions

- Provide information about incidents to unauthorized persons or agencies

## SUMMARY AND REVIEW

1. What is the most important thing to remember when you answer the telephone in the communications center?

2. List ten responsibilities of the medical dispatcher. Do medical communicators have additional roles and responsibilities in your system?

3. List the range of services or levels of care available to the public through your system.

4. What would you do if the power to your communications center failed?

5. What is the availability of mutual aid or other outside resources in your service area? Do you have clear guidelines in place to tell you when to use mutual aid resources?

6. What type of quality assurance plan does your system provide for medical communicators? What about for field care-givers?

7. List five activities inappropriate to the medical dispatcher. Do the policies and procedures in place in your system allow any of these activities to occur regularly?

# Chapter 6

# BASIC COMMUNICATION AND TELECOMMUNICTION THEORY

*"MedStar, where do you need us?"*
— standard phrasing used when
answering emergency phone lines
for MedStar Ambulance, Fort Worth, Texas

*"MedStar, may I help you?"*
— standard phrasing used when
answering nonemergency phone lines

*"MedStar, can you help us?"*
— SSC answering emergency phone line
during first training shift

## THE FOUR COMPONENTS OF COMMUNICATION

What is communication? Most simply defined, *communication is the act of making contact with the mind of another person.*

How is this achieved? Communication can be divided into two broad categories: The use of facial expressions, gestures, or other bodily signals; and the use of language. *Language itself is used in four basic ways: reading, writing, speaking, and listening.* Some individuals can be observed to do these things better than others, whether through innate talent or through training or both.

## TRAINING VERSUS NATURAL TALENT

You were taught to read, first identifying single letters, then words, and then associating ideas with combinations of words. You learned to write in much the same way, by observing successful writing and then imitating the results.

You were taught to speak, in that you learned to mimic words as a baby and then learned the rules of grammar in school; but what type of training did you receive in how to communicate a specific idea?

Some individuals may have native endowments that enable them to become better speakers than others, but training is required to bring those talents into full bloom. Likewise, skill in listening is either a native gift, or it must be acquired by training.

The general assumption that the ability to speak well and to listen well is a natural gift for which no training is required is an amazing assumption. The fact that this assumption is widely held is reflected in the manner in which we receive (or do *not* receive) our training in these areas during the course of our schooling.

Listening as a skill is learned first and used most in the course of one's life (approximately 46 percent of the time).[1] Of the four communications skills (reading, writing, speaking, and listening), listening is the least taught throughout all the years of schooling.

Speaking is learned next, and is used 30 percent of the time. As a skill, speaking remains almost as untaught as listening.

Reading is learned next, used 15 percent of the time, and is taught less than writing.

Writing is learned last, used the least (9 percent), and receives more instruction time than any other communications skill.

## IF I CAN SPEAK ENGLISH, HOW HARD CAN THIS BE?

Effective speaking and listening, the two generally untaught skills, are generally much more difficult to perfect than reading and writing, in which we do receive instruction.

At first glance, it would appear that speaking and listening perfectly parallel writing and reading. Both pairs involve the use of language where one mind reaches out and another responds.

If you can write well, why should it be any more difficult for you to communicate easily via the spoken word? If you can read easily, and comprehend and understand the information you read, then why is it not equally as easy for you to listen, understand, and retain words that are spoken to you? The act of mastering speaking and listening skills is more difficult than reading and writing because of the differences in speed and the transitory nature of the exchanges.

If you read something and don't understand it, you can read it again. If you write something and realize it doesn't exactly get your message across, you can rewrite it again and again until you get it right.

Speaking, especially in the context of our jobs as medical communicators, is like a performance that, once given, cannot be improved. It can be improved *upon* in a later performance, but that one performance must be *as good as it can possibly be*. Once the curtain goes down, it is finished—unchangeable. You may be able to do a better job at a later time, but on a particular occasion, *whatever excellence you are able to achieve must be achieved right then and there*. Your listening skills function in much the same way.

---

[1] Mortimer J. Adler, *How to Speak, How to Listen*, Macmillan Publishing Co., Inc., 1983.

Another reason speaking and listening are more difficult than reading and writing is that the mechanics of the actions differ. Reading and writing, though important skills, can be done separately, and usually are. Speaking and listening, especially in the context of our jobs, must be performed simultaneously. We play the roles of both speaker and listener at once. The art of giving a prepared speech, where you are allowed to move from introduction to conclusion without interruption, can be learned without mastering the skill of listening. Silent, passive listening can be dealt with without perfecting speaking skills.

Your position as a medical communicator requires that you achieve excellence in clear, directed speaking *and* open, retentive listening, *both individually and simultaneously.*

## BEHAVIOR MODIFICATION TECHNIQUES

If you are training for a position as a medical communicator, then you are chronologically an adult. You have had many years to build a multitude of speaking and listening habits, both good and bad. The first step to mastering basic communications skills is to identify these habits.

### Poor Listening Habits

These are the five most commonly encountered *bad* listening habits:

- Paying more attention to the speaker's speech mannerisms and/or attitude than to the substance of what is being said
- Giving the appearance of listening while allowing your attention to wander
- Allowing distractions to divert your attention from the speaker
- Reacting and/or overreacting to certain words or phrases that happen to arouse adverse emotional responses, so that you are then predisposed in your assessment of what the speaker is actually saying
- Allowing an initial lack of interest to prevent you from hearing the speaker's explanation of what is actually happening

Stop now and think: How many of these bad habits do you have? Now that these bad habits have been identified, you must consciously and conscientiously work to improve your listening skills. The fastest and easiest way to rid yourself of bad habits is to replace them with good ones.

### Positive Listening Habits

Here are some *good* listening habits that should become automatic for you:

- Have at least the intellectual courtesy to initially assume that everything the speaker says is important enough for you to pay attention.
- Make sure that your mind is actively engaged in listening.
- Concentrate; pay attention.
- Form a mental picture from what the speaker says.
- Do not allow your perceptions to be clouded by any irrelevant emotional response you might have to the speaker's tone of voice or speech mannerisms.
- The mental effort you expend must be equal to the task set by the difficulty or complexity of what the speaker is saying.
- Penetrate through the words to the thought that lies behind them.
- Overcome and adjust for the differences in vocabulary between you and the speaker.
- Pick out the most important parts of what the speaker is saying. While everything the speaker says will be important in the right context, not everything said will be critical to patient care or crew safety. Highlight the most important words in your mind.
- Remember that your time with the speaker is finite. *Saying exactly what you mean is one of the hardest things in the world to do. Listening to what others say in order to determine what they mean is equally as difficult.*

Improved Speaking Habits

Once you have begun to improve your listening skills, you should be able to work at perfecting your speaking skills at the same time. These are some excellent speaking skills to cultivate:

- Plan in advance exactly what you will say, and then stick to it. Improvise only when you have to.
- While a conversation is taking place, don't listen only to yourself. Change gears when the speaker begins to respond to what you have said, and really listen.
- When you are asked a question, make the effort to understand it *before* you answer it. Make sure you know exactly what is being asked before you respond.
- When you ask a question, make sure it is clearly understood. Don't assume that the other person understands what you mean. Be prepared to ask the question a number of different ways until you are sure it is understood.
- Interrupt the speaker only if:
    - the need to gain immediate control of the conversation exists
    - the speaker's hysteria threshold must be broken before pertinent information can be obtained
    - the situation is time-critical
- Do not engage in noncritical side conversations if the speaker can

hear them. If your telephone microphone is muted, then you may alert your partners to an incoming call or advise your partners of critical patient status, scene hazards, special patient needs, and so on.

## THE CHALLENGE OF A NEW PERSPECTIVE

So you made it through EMT school with no prior medical experience. You took a job for very little money in a field that horrified your parents and disgusted your friends. You ran transfers until you thought you'd lose your mind. Then you enrolled in paramedic school; you stumbled through nearly the entire course before it started to make sense to you, but you survived and graduated. After many lonely meals, you learned not to discuss your work at the dinner table. You are employed by an innovative EMS service on the cutting edge of modern technology and with a nationwide reputation for excellence. You are certified in Advanced Cardiac Life Support and Pre-Hospital Trauma Life Support. You passed the National Registry Examination with flying colors. You keep your CPR Instructor status current. You know your service area like the back of your hand, and you can work a full arrest in your sleep. Congratulations. Now try to do your job blindfolded and with both hands tied behind your back.

The process of achieving excellence as a medical communicator will teach you many things that are not obviously encompassed by the job itself. You will discover that people are both stronger and more fragile than you ever imagined. You will find that you are capable of almost limitless patience. You will learn to listen to six different conversations at once, and understand them all. Suddenly, after weeks of frustration, you will realize that you can listen to the sounds of one event taking place, talk about a second, and watch a third, while entering into the computer information about a fourth and separate occurrence. You will discover that human behavior, even in reaction to a crisis situation, forms patterns that can, with experience, be anticipated and planned for. You will learn that delivering a planned response works better than making it up as you go. And, finally, you will understand that while to err may be human, there are two basic kinds of mistakes: those that are unavoidable, and those that, with care, practice, and planning, could have been averted altogether.

## COMMUNICATION VERSUS TELECOMMUNICATION

What's the difference between simple communication and telecommunication? Easy answer, right? *Telecommunication is communication accomplished through the use of an electronic audio and/or visual link.* This is a legitimate definition of the word. For our more specific purposes, our most critical telecommunication takes place over a telephone line. The big difference between face-to-face conversation and our use of telecommunication is both simple and profound: *The person with whom you are attempting to communicate, who is depending on you for total support and direction, and on whom you are depending to obtain life-saving information and to perform life-saving techniques, CANNOT SEE YOU.*

How important can that difference be? As you will learn, the scope of that difference and the medical call-taker's ability to bridge the existing gap can and frequently do mean literally the difference between life and death.

## WORKING WITH A HANDICAP

If you have never functioned with or in spite of a physical handicap, this will be a learning experience for you. To understand how to compensate for the absence of direct vision when performing the medical communicator's duties, first you must understand what is actually impaired by the handicap.

Each person who communicates with you, whether by radio or by telephone, wants, needs, and expects certain things from you, whether or not they are able to verbalize those desires and expectations. The field crews who talk to you on a radio channel want clear, concise, usable information. They expect you to perform your job duties with an extraordinarily high level of accuracy. In fact, they expect your performance to be flawless. They expect you to be professional at all times. *Field personnel who discuss this point openly with you will admit that the communicator who does not display professional radio behavior embarrasses them.* They need to feel total confidence in your abilities. They need, in order to perform their own jobs well, to know that you are calm, assured, and in total control of the system.

The caller who accesses the system by telephone has even higher expectations and operates under an even greater disadvantage. The field paramedic or EMT usually knows you; if she/he doesn't know you well, you have usually at least met. The field crew member can see a picture of you in her/his mind. If you haven't met, the field crews at least feel some degree of identification with you, since you work for the same system and they are acquainted with your procedures.

Private citizens who call for help usually do so completely uninformed. They may expect you, first of all, to simply do what they tell you to do ("Just send the damned ambulance!"). They definitely want you to remain calm and courteous, even when they become hostile or abusive. They want the ambulance to arrive immediately. Some callers expect you to tell them what to do until the ambulance arrives; with the advent of the 9-1-1 system, this expectation has become dramatically more frequent. Some callers honestly don't know specifically what they want from you; they just want their problem to be solved, and they want it solved *right now.* Since they don't know how to resolve the problem, that becomes your job. Whether it is verbalized or not, each and every caller wants, needs, expects, and deserves to draw from you confidence, comfort and reassurance.

## THE SPOKEN WORD VERSUS GESTURE

Pay attention. This is the single most important fact to remember about telecommunication. *Gesture is embedded in language.*

Try this: Stand in front of a mirror. Now smile. Think of something sweet and warm and funny. Stand there and keep at it until you are really smiling, even with your eyes. Now say to your image in the mirror, as seriously as you know how, "You are pond scum. You disgust me. You are repulsive. YOU MAKE ME SICK." Didn't work well, did it? Try the reverse. Standing in front of the mirror, picture in your mind someone you really, really despise. Let your feelings show on your face. Scowl. Frown. Get the image solidly in your mind, and then say very sweetly, "You're wonderful, and I love you very much." If you seriously try to do this, you will quickly see that it simply doesn't work. *Certain facial expressions and body gestures are programmed into our brains to equate with certain emotions.*

When we are very young, we acquire understanding and communications skills through *observation and imitation*. We observe that certain emotions are accompanied by specific body language, and we learn to imitate the display process. As we observe the same pairing of gesture and emotion again and again, a connection is formed in our brains that recognizes the relationship and stores the information for future reference. How can we unconsciously recognize this abstract connection? As facial expressions and body gestures change, the pronunciation and delivery of the spoken word changes. The actual wave form of the sound is changed, and we unconsciously register and interpret that change.

If, as you listen to a client complain over a telephone line, you mute your microphone, roll your eyes, and comment to your partners, "Yeah, yeah, yeah...," the next words that you say to the caller will reflect the emotions of impatience and disgust. The sound waves created when the words "Yes, ma'am" are spoken first by a supportive, caring speaker and then by an inattentive, bored speaker are different. On some level, the caller will recognize the difference. While the caller's reaction to your tone of voice may not always erupt into a verbal confrontation, your ability to direct and control the conversation for the good of the patient will be diminished.

Some of our reactions to vocal inflections may very well be instinctive; if they are, then no amount of behavior modification will change the manner in which we react. How much of this de-coding process is instinctive and how much is learned behavior is still under debate.

By a perverse quirk of nature, it is much more difficult to "charge" your speaking voice with an emotion you do not feel than it is to disguise an emotion you do feel. While some speakers can be trained to hide anger or impatience from a listener who cannot see them, most have real difficulty projecting a caring attitude if they truly do not care. Even when your motivation is appropriate, you will usually have to exaggerate the positive emotion in your voice for the caller to interpret it clearly, and without error.

## THE NATURE OF THE MEDICAL COMMUNICATOR

Why did you originally choose emergency medical service as a career? Since our industry is only now beginning to offer wages comparable to other business classifications, we can safely assume that it wasn't for the money. Some will say it was the excitement that drew them, and for some that continues to be a factor. EMS personnel, as a whole, have an interesting self-image. We see ourselves as stronger and tougher than the average person; we can cope with anything. Most of us are very reluctant to talk about emotions and values; we talk instead about "good calls," where the patient was critically ill or injured. If you could convince a cross section of EMS personnel to do some basic, totally honest self-evaluation and *then to honestly and openly verbalize the results*, you would find that the vast majority of those personnel have one thing in common: They want to help, and because they have discovered strengths within themselves that allow them to function during crisis situations better than the average person, they feel obligated to do so. This is the primary motivation that the medical dispatcher *must* feel. If you do not genuinely care about our field crews and those who call for our help, you will not be capable of performing this job satisfactorily, because you will not be able to consistently fake it for long periods of time. If your head's not right, it just won't work.

## SUMMARY AND REVIEW

1. What is communication?

2. What are the four components of communication?

3. List five poor listening habits. Now play back the videotape in your head. How many of these have you been guilty of committing?

4. List what you believe are the five most effective ways to improve your listening skills. Keep a record for one week of how often you use these behavior modification techniques. What percentage do you believe your performance has improved? 50 percent? 100 percent?

5. How can you improve your speaking habits?

6. Why are speaking and listening such difficult skills to learn?

7. What is telecommunication?

8. What are the important differences between communication and telecommunication?

9. What is the most important thing to remember about gesture?

10. What steps can you take to overcome the handicaps of not having visual contact with the caller?

# Chapter 7

# BASIC TELEPHONE TECHNIQUES

*"I will be the pattern of all patience."*
— *William Shakespeare,* King Lear

## THE TELEPHONE AS A TOOL

In both the private and public sectors of our industry, *unbelievable amounts of business and good will are thrown away each year because of the way customers and clients are treated during telephone interactions. Thrown-away business and good will mean decreased customer satisfaction and decreased system revenues. Decreased customer satisfaction equals decreased job security; decreased system revenues equals inferior equipment, fewer benefits, and smaller and less frequent salary increases.* Good telephone etiquette is a skill every medical communicator must master.

Remember, humans interpret many behavior patterns as attacks; basically, an attack is anything that prevents us from getting what we want. How do humans respond to real or imagined attacks? Repeat this several times: *Attack, counterattack; Escape, pursuit.*

## THE FIVE THINGS YOU SHOULD NEVER SAY TO A CUSTOMER

There are five phrases that are virtually guaranteed to be viewed as attacks by the caller. These simply *must* be avoided.

These five phrases must *never, never, never* be spoken to a client or customer. Familiarize yourself with them; then *don't ever use them again.*

- *"I don't know."* Get with the program. *Never* admit to *anyone* that you don't know anything, even when you don't. A frequently heard variation of "I don't know" is "I just got here." Again, grow up. Nobody cares. Instead, say, "Let me check on that for you."
- *"Hang on just a second, I'll be right back."* While this is certainly friendly and familiar, it's just not very professional. If you could survey a cross section of your customers, I'd be willing to bet the farm on the fact that, given the choice between friendly and professional, they would choose professional every time. We don't install garage door-openers for a living; we provide patient care and transportation. Replace the previous phrase with, "I'll need to put you on hold for a minute. Is that all right?" This gives the caller the feeling that she/he is in control; it magnifies any attempt you make to satisfy the caller's need. Remember the caller's name, and state your own. Then, when you pick up the phone again, begin the conversation with, Hello, Mrs. Smith. This is Jane again...."
- *"You'll have to...."* Never, never tell a caller what she or he has to do. Your customers don't *have* to do anything. Instead, say, "Let me give you another number to call," or "Here's how we can handle that. Please call....."
- *"We can't (or don't, or won't) do that."* Instead, offer another solution. Another very effective tool is to become the "phantom supervisor." All it takes to make this work is a commitment on your part to take *total responsibility* for the problem, and to come up with a resolution. The caller feels important, because she/he is receiving personalized attention. You feel good because you have successfully dealt with a difficult situation. Just take the caller's name and number, and offer yours. Then say, "Let me see what I can do; I'll call you right back." This type of personal investment not only gives the caller an obvious "pat"; it leads you to think more creatively and try harder to find a solution to the problem. Now it's not just the system's credibility that's on the line; it's yours.
- *"No......"* *Never* begin a sentence with a negative (unless, of course, it's to sing a chorus of "Nobody knows the trouble I've seen," which is appropriate in any high-volume dispatch center whenever you are not actively talking on the phone or the radio). Starting with a negative is invariably seen as an attack by the caller, and predictable defensive behavior (counterattack, escape) will follow.

After you've practiced and perfected these techniques, you will find that dealing with people over the telephone becomes a kind of game; a serious game, to be sure, but a game nevertheless. The object of the game is to win. You win by projecting a positive attitude, controlling your temper, and satisfying the needs of your customers so they can't complain any more.

## BASIC TELEPHONE TECHNIQUES

There are three basic skills involved in working with the telephone that are so simple, their value seems patently obvious. However, simple ideas are often both the most profound and the most easily missed, so I will outline them for you here.

The first, often unconsidered element that will affect the final outcome of a situation involving a call for help is *the speed with which you answer the telephone.*

## THE SPEED OF THE RESPONSE: FIRST IMPRESSIONS COUNT

The first consideration in answering the telephone is the speed with which you answer. The importance of this one factor is frequently overlooked by beginning SSCs.

People call the communications center because they need emergency help. As they dial the phone, they are also dealing with a multitude of doubts about the situation and about the system as a whole: "Will he die? Will the person who answers the telephone at 9-1-1 know what to do? Will someone come to help me? Is there anything else I should be doing? Will the system work for me?" The longer that telephone rings without being answered, the more time exists for the caller's doubts to grow and multiply until they are completely out of control. Answer the telephone within an absolute maximum of two rings. The impression created when you answer quickly is that of a sharp, attentive, concerned professional.

Many different types of nonemergency calls are also received in the dispatch center; each of these callers will have a different mind-set. While the speed with which you answer their calls may or may not directly and immediately affect patient care, it will very definitely affect the caller's impression of and level of confidence in you, your department, and your system as a whole. *If a need did not exist, the caller would not have dialed your telephone number. Whatever motivated the caller to place that call is the most important thing to her/him at that moment. Your job is to satisfy the needs of those who call for your help or service. Answer the telephone in two rings or less.*

If the caller is the transfer coordinator for a local hospital, imagine what her/his mind-set is:

> "Busy...overworked...nobody called to schedule this transfer...I asked them to do it yesterday...the appointment is for seven-thirty...it's seven-fifteen now...she's going to be late...the doctor's office will call and bitch...my boss is going to kill me...."

The longer the caller has to wait for the telephone to be answered, the more time negative thoughts and impressions have to build. *Answer the telephone in two rings or less.*

If the caller is a customer with a question or complaint about a bill, what thoughts do you suppose are running through her/his head? Again, imagine the mind-set:

> "I'm seventy-seven years old...my Social Security check is only $408.00 a month...this bill is for $450.00...how will I ever pay this?...I've paid my bills on time all my life...it was only a nonemergency transfer...this price is outrageous...what am I going to do?...."

The longer that phone rings, the more time the caller's frustration has to grow. *Answer the telephone in two rings or less.*

Whether the caller is a field crew member who is hungry or a hospital administrator advising of a hospital status change, the caller believes the call is important; otherwise they would not have dialed the telephone. *Answer the telephone in two rings or less.*

## COMMUNICATIONS CENTER OVERLOAD

In any truly progressive system, staffing levels in the dispatch center are planned and schedules established to staff at higher levels when the call demand is high. However, even with responsible management, there will always be times when more telephone lines are ringing than can be immediately answered. This is a situation of *overload*. Even careful planning cannot eliminate all occurrences of overload. Overload happens most commonly in high-performance systems where the communicators give pre-arrival instructions. As you receive call information for a critical situation that demands pre-arrival instructions, you are ideally unavailable to take further calls until the critical situation is resolved.

When overload occurs, you must *reprioritize your job tasks* constantly. Here are some general guidelines to help you in the reprioritization process:

- Answer the emergency lines first.
- Watch carefully to avoid entering duplicate calls (in situations involving major accidents with multiple injuries, explosions, etc., you may receive multiple telephone notifications of the event).
- Prepare to switch roles with your partner(s); if she/he is working as radio operator and is caught on a telephone line, answer the radio until she/he is free. If you have entered a call and see that your partner is involved in a complicated call-taking process or in the process of giving pre-arrival instructions, avoid dispatch delays by pre-alerting and/or dispatching the response yourself.
- If more emergency lines are ringing than you can answer and still give pre-arrival instructions, tell the callers in critical situations that you are going to dispatch the ambulance *now*; tell them that you will now place them on hold while you dispatch the paramedics and that you will then pick up the telephone and tell them what to do. Remind them both not to hang up, and that the paramedics are on their way.
- Answer the nonemergency lines after the emergency lines have been answered. *Be very wary of answering a nonemergency line,*

*snapping, "Hold please," and placing the caller immediately on hold.* While, in any system, specific telephone lines are usually designated as emergency and nonemergency numbers, callers frequently either dial the wrong number by mistake, dial the only number they can find, or have an entirely different perception of "emergency" than we do. *While we may have in place comprehensive, detailed procedures, there is never any guarantee that the caller has read the book*

- When you *must* place a caller on hold, do so politely (it is always preferable to ask, "Can you hold, please?").
- Answer any lines on hold as quickly as you can. When you pick up on the line, begin by saying, "I'm sorry to have kept you waiting. This is John, may I help you?"
- Answer any administrative or private lines last. Calls that are administrative in nature can wait. First, answer all calls that could possibly be emergencies or involve direct voice contact with clients.
- As soon as the activity level will allow, prepare to make whatever follow-up calls are necessary. If the 9-1-1 lines all ring at once, you may sometimes disconnect to prevent additional callers from receiving a busy signal. Also, you may receive requests for dispatch which later require additional data. In these cases, the caller must be recontacted for further information.
- Have a plan in place that tells you what to do if the overload conditions persist. *Remember, in a crisis a planned response is always better than an unplanned response.* If you schedule single-person shifts, know who your back-up should be, and know where they are and how to contact them at all times.

## ANSWERING THE EMERGENCY TELEPHONE LINE

One of the first things you should learn about answering any telephone line in a medical communications center is to *keep your phrasing short.* Have you ever considered just how irritating it is to people who are impatient or in a hurry (like me) to call a business and have a person who sounds like she may be all of fourteen years old say, "G-o-o-o-o-o-d morning! Greater North American Wonderful Widgets Incorporated, Marketing Division, Customer Service Department, this is Courtney speaking, may I help you?" *Courtney*, huh? Well, I'll tell you something. I didn't dial this phone number to hear *Courtney* talk. I called so *Courtney* could listen to *me* talk. Please, please, for the sake of people like me who live their entire lives in a hurry, keep your greeting *short and to the point.*

Many different answering techniques for emergency telephone lines have been tested throughout the country. A wise choice to implement as procedure is the one technique that has met with the most widespread success. One very effective phrase to use is, "Acme Ambulance, where do you need us?"

Okay, okay. If you've never used this answering technique before, you're going to feel pretty silly the first few times you try it. However, this is an important procedure to have in place in your communications department, *because it works*. It quickly accomplishes the task the communicator will try to achieve first: *The identification of the location where the response is needed.*

How does it work? First, it cuts down on unnecessary time waste in a time-critical situation. If you answer the telephone saying, "Acme," or "Ambulance," only one thing is obvious to the caller: she/he has dialed the correct phone number. When you ask, "Where do you need us?", it establishes several things in the mind of the caller.

This technique lets the caller know that you *are* Acme Ambulance Service, and that *you already understand that the caller needs your help*. You *already* know the call is not in reference to a bill or a simple request for information. It also gives the caller immediate reassurance of a sort, because the phrasing is short and very directed. You are established as the professional who knows exactly what she/he is doing.

By using this technique, *you force the caller to focus on a single piece of information*. The address or the incident location is the first of three critical units of information (the incident address, the call-back number, and the initial presumptive patient condition category) that must be obtained before you can pre-alert or dispatch the response. By immediately demanding this information, you can frequently stop the initial hysterical outbreak, or avoid it altogether. You have given yourself an immediate psychological edge.

## ANSWERING THE NON-EMERGENCY TELEPHONE LINE

There are many appropriate ways in which to answer a non-emergency telephone line in the communications center. One method commonly used is, "Acme Ambulance, may I help you?"

The most important consideration in completing this task is to *initiate the conversation with a positive, professional, caring attitude*. An even more positive phrase to use is, "Acme Ambulance, how may I help you?" Of *course* you can help her; that's why she called your number. Asking *how* you can help immediately places you in a position of control. Again, it will frequently be necessary to exaggerate the inflection in your voice to make sure your message is clear.

Answering the telephone in a positive, energetic manner gives you another immediate psychological edge. If you answer in a neutral tone, or your voice reflects your desire to hurry up and get this over with, you have unknowingly communicated a weakness. The caller who is also on edge and is having a bad day will, on some level, interpret this as a signal to attack. If you answer in a positive, "upbeat" manner, you are perceived as strong. The caller will frequently assume that whatever problems exist lie with her or him, and not with you.

"Psych up" before you answer each telephone call. A positive attitude should be projected each time you contact a client. Remember the motivation and mind-set of the caller; remember that yours is a service organization, and that you can only continue to provide that service through the good will of your clients.

## HANDLING COMPLAINTS

Taking complaint information can also become a game, if you can depersonalize the process enough to play. There are two important points to remember when preparing to deal with customer complaints:

- First, customer satisfaction is a hundred small things done well; and
- Second, every complaint is an opportunity to convert a nonbeliever.

When you answer the phone and the caller says, "I want to file a complaint," the dispatcher's first task is clear. In any medical care and transportation system, you must first identify the type of complaint. Is the problem with the attitude of a field crew? If so, the information must be relayed to a field supervisor. Is the complaint about patient care? This type of complaint should be relayed to the clinical coordinator, the training director, the medical director, the field supervisor, or all of the above. Is the caller angry about the treatment she/he received when calling the dispatch center? If so, the grievance must be referred to the communications manager.

In some instances, it is interesting to allow yourself to be used as a "fire wall" for the appropriate manager. You may politely ask, "Could you tell me a little about the problem, so I will know which division manager in our system should be notified?" Then brace yourself, because most of the time, you will get blasted. However, consider this: if someone sneaks up behind you and jabs a finger between your ribs, you will scream and jump. If you know it's coming, you can sit still and maintain a neutral expression, because you were prepared for the action. If you have invited a negative type of interaction with a client, or have asked for it, your own subconscious will not interpret it as an attack; you will be able to handle it graciously.

People don't reason well when they're extremely angry; if you can take the abuse, try letting the caller go crazy on you *before* she/he talks to the appropriate supervisory contact. *Never* make excuses, or try to justify the offending behavior or event. Use neutral words and sounds to encourage the caller to let off some steam. The caller will feel calmer after venting. You will be able to relay some details about the problem to the manager who will be returning the complainant's call. The manager involved will then be at least partially prepared for the ensuing conversation. With a little effort on your part, the situation will be somewhat improved *before the caller ever makes the official complaint.*

When dealing with a complaint, even if the caller's attitude becomes hostile or abusive, do not answer with discourteous or unpleasant behavior. Take the caller's name and number and have the appropriate supervisory or management person make the subsequent contact and attempt to resolve the problem.

Again, this type of normally hostile interaction can become a game. How do you win? The winner continues to use courteous behavior even when the hostile caller does not, controls her/his temper when others cannot, provides a measure of customer satisfaction when others could not, and hands a manager or administrator a neatly tied package of information enabling her/him to more easily and comfortably deal with an unpleasant situation.

## A NOTE ABOUT EVALUATIONS

Although routine, regularly scheduled performance evaluations should be performed every six months after a medical communicator has completed training and been assigned to a position, other performance reviews called *interim evaluations* should be performed by the communications manager frequently and regularly. These written evaluations should note compliance with and deviations from departmental procedures and standards for telephone and radio behavior. Information from these interim evaluations can then be used to compile the general evaluation performed every six months. *On every interim performance evaluation sheet, the phrasing used to answer specific telephone lines should be noted.*

## DON'T HANG UP!

The final basic component of effective telecommunication in emergency medical service is this: *Don't hang up the phone.*

For years, the EMS dispatcher was allowed and even encouraged to follow her/his most basic instinct: *if the telephone conversation becomes unpleasant, hang up.* (When I began training in EMS communications in 1982, I was told: "If a caller *ever* curses at you on the telephone, immediately disconnect them.") When the dispatcher answered the telephone, the person calling might be angry, abusive, or hysterical. The feelings left with the dispatcher after these calls were negative. The most obvious solution to this problem was to hang up the phone, as quickly as possible. *Escape, pursuit, escape.* An absolute minimum of dispatch information was obtained very quickly, and the telephone call was terminated.

Now that we understand more about the psychology of the human response to crisis (whether real or perceived), we have also come to realize that amazing things can be accomplished, if you simply *don't hang up the phone.*

Hysterical callers who have witnessed the cardiac arrest of a loved one can be taught to perform life-saving CPR. Small children who have limited vocabularies can be persuaded to give valuable information. Third-party callers who think they have no information to give can be directed to assist in the call-prioritization process. Incredibly angry citizens with service complaints can have their anger completely defused, and can be left with the belief that your system does, indeed, employ wonderful, professional, compassionate people.

Especially during the initial phases of training, the impulse to terminate an unpleasant conversation can be very strong. *A good rule to use is this: Don't end a telephone conversation until you (or another SSC on duty, or the communications administrator) have changed the attitude of the caller or the projected outcome of the incident from the negative to the positive.* Occasionally with nonemergency callers, you will find yourself in a situation where *everything* you say and every approach you try seems to make things worse. On those rare occasions, it may be best to take call-back information, terminate the conversation, and have someone else return the call.

## SUMMARY AND REVIEW

1. What impact can your telephone conversational skills have on the eventual success or failure of your system or your company?

2. What are the five things you should never say to a customer on the telephone?

3. List the three basic principles of successfully dealing with the telephone caller.

4. Practice preparing for communications center overload. Sit with a partner or as a group. Have each person in the group write out a scenario for a certain time period in the communications center. Note how many calls are received, what type of calls they are, and how many units are available in the system. Now trade scenarios with another person. How would you reprioritize the tasks in your scenario?

5. How are emergency and nonemergency telephone lines answered in your system? How could your answering techniques be improved?

# Chapter 8

# TELEPHONE TRIAGE AND REMOTE INTERVENTION

*"Now, listen, here, Miss Priss. My doctor has all that information, and I don't believe that I need to answer any more of your nosy little questions. You just hang up this phone and send the ambulance to my house RIGHT THIS MINUTE." (Disconnect.)*
— *Elderly female requesting ambulance service in Fort Worth, Texas, in April 1988*

*"Lady, you don't have the sense God gave a pissant."*
— *Male requesting ambulance service in Fort Worth, Texas, in November 1987*

## WHAT IS TELEPHONE TRIAGE?

Telephone triage is the process of asking planned, structured questions of a caller requesting medical assistance, and then analyzing the responses to those questions to determine the needs of the caller and the patient. When those needs have been clearly identified, the process of priority dispatching can begin.

## PRIORITY DISPATCHING DEFINED

Priority dispatching is the process by which medical communicators, having received specialized training, use standardized telephone triage interviewing protocols to prioritize requests for medical assistance according to existing needs. The goal is to send the minimum number of personnel in the safest response mode that will satisfy all the needs of the patient and ensure the delivery of the highest quality patient care. When the process is complete and/or a portion of the process is handed off to another medical communicator, the process of administering remote intervention can begin, where appropriate.

## WHAT IS REMOTE INTERVENTION?

Remote intervention consists of directions given to callers by trained medical communicators. These instructions are delivered with these goals in mind:

- To provide life-saving intervention in cases of critical trauma or illness, thereby slowing or completely arresting the death process
- To prevent further harm, damage, or injury to the patient, thereby improving the quality of her/his life following the incident
- To ensure the safety of the caller
- To narrow the time gap between when the call for help is made and when the care-givers arrive on the scene
- To provide control of the scene until the care-givers arrive
- To provide the caller the opportunity to do everything possible for the patient while awaiting the arrival of the care-givers, thus minimizing the psychological damage to the caller upon termination of the incident

## THE PHILOSOPHY BEHIND THE CHANGE

With the exception of the last eight to ten years, dispatching in emergency medical service has traditionally been a relatively simple, uncomplicated task. The minimum amount of information needed to initiate the response was gathered, and the maximum response was always sent. More and louder must be better, right? With the advent of more sophisticated guidelines for field care of the sick and injured, we discovered that the maximum response was *not* always in the patient's best interest. We acknowledged that the act of endangering both responders and bystanders during a medically unnecessary emergency response was both irresponsible and unacceptable. We recognized the needs of our own field employees, and the need to keep our organization financially sound if we are to be able to provide those employees with the salary structure, state-of-the-art equipment, and benefits they so obviously deserve. *We realized that the medical communicator was no longer forced to accept the role of the helpless bystander, but could and must take an active part in administering patient care.*

## COMMON OBJECTIONS AND MISCONCEPTIONS

The medical communicator must understand the basic philosophy of telephone triage in order to be an effective and consistent medical dispatcher.

These are the five most commonly held *misconceptions* about the use of telephone triage interviewing techniques:

- The caller is too upset to respond accurately
- The caller doesn't know the required information.
- The medical expertise of the call-taker is not important.
- The SSC is too busy to waste time asking questions, giving instructions, or following specific questioning formats.

- Telephone instructions from medical communicators cannot help victims and may even be dangerous.

The first two items in the previous list are deeply ingrained in the minds of some field paramedics and experienced dispatchers. However, they are *misconceptions*; they are simply not true. Medical dispatch experts have shown that through proper techniques and the use of interrogation protocols, significantly more vital information can be obtained than when other traditional methods are used.

In response systems where telephone triage and priority dispatch training are not provided, call-takers often respond to the unpleasant, uncooperative, or hysterical caller by obtaining the location of the incident and the basic nature only, thereby missing or failing to recognize a possibly critical situation.

It is critically important that you learn and use the techniques detailed in this text. *If you don't know the right questions to ask, you can't get the right answers.* Until you learn to utilize standard formats and calming techniques to break through the "hysteria threshold," you can't be in control of the call-taking procedure.

## CALL PRIORITIZATION VERSUS CALL SCREENING

In any responsible EMS system, the medical communicators *prioritize* calls; *they do not screen them*. *Prioritization* allows the sending of the minimum number of personnel in the safest response mode to address all the patient's needs. *Screening* implies or denotes the practice of referring noncritical or undesirable calls to another agency, or otherwise not sending an ambulance when a response is requested. *Never, never, never, never refuse to send an ambulance when a response is requested in your service area or in an area covered by mutual aid contracts. Always, always, always, always send an ambulance when such a request is made.*

## PRACTICAL GUIDELINES FOR ESTABLISHING ALGORITHMS

Algorithms differ slightly with each system and each service area. Although the medical treatment and intervention principles remain basically the same nationwide, local custom and preference should always be taken into account. If medical priority dispatch is not common in your area, or if your system is just beginning the process of defining standardized algorithms, you need to know some practical, workable steps to complete the process.

These elements should be considered in any system as telephone prioritization and pre-arrival algorithms are established:

- First, research the project thoroughly. Make some phone calls of your own; if you don't know anyone who works in an EMS system in another part of the state or the country, pick a city and call directory assistance. Then call the nonemergency number for the private provider or city service that provides ambulance service for that area. Ask for the communications supervisor or the clinical coordinator, and explain, over and over, who you are and what you want. Eventually, you'll connect with the person who can give you the information you need. Ask what telephone standards they use, and ask them to send you copies of their formats.

- Compare the information you receive with that contained in *Principles of Emergency Medical Dispatch* by Clawson and Dernecoeur (they were the originators of the concept). What type of system are the protocols to be used in? Is it single- or multi-tiered? How can you adapt algorithms in use in other systems to meet your own needs?

- Be careful not to strike out too hastily into territory that is completely untried. If you deviate too far from established procedures, you're leaving yourself vulnerable to attack in the form of civil litigation.

- Present your suggestions for algorithm structure, along with your research materials, to your clinical coordinator, medical director, and physician advisory group. This is an important step. Do you want to end up on a witness stand somewhere trying to explain what degree of medical expertise qualifies you to initiate the use of these protocols? Probably not. Pass the responsibility for the final medical decisions to people who have "M.D." or "D.O." after their names.

- Make arrangements to have the protocol information displayed in an easy-to-use format in your communications center: in your CAD system, in a manual card file, whatever. It's important that your medical dispatchers don't initially try to rely on memory; remember how unreliable our memories are. Follow the protocols, exactly as they were approved by your medical advisors, every time you use them.

- Provide training for communicators, field employees, first responders, fire departments, police departments, or any other agency or group that might make scene responses with your units. It's important for everyone to understand the benefits of this system and exactly how it works.

- Conduct a public education campaign (this should be done periodically even in systems where the process is already in place). People who are unaware that they will be asked 20 questions when they call for an ambulance response can become very hostile very quickly.

- Make conforming with the accepted protocols part of your evaluation and quality assurance process.

- Review the protocols regularly, at least once yearly. Submit written suggestions for change and improvement to your medical advisors for their approval.

## SUMMARY AND REVIEW

1. Define telephone triage.
2. Define priority dispatching.
3. Define remote intervention.
4. What are some common objections to the practice of telephone triage?
5. What is the difference between call prioritization and call screening?
6. Are telephone algorithms in place in your system? Are they in use? Who wrote them?

# Chapter 9

# ADVANCED TELECOMMUNICATIONS TECHNIQUES

*"What did he say?"*
— *Former President Ronald Reagan to his wife, Nancy*

## FIRST, LEARN THE BASICS

Once you have begun to master basic telecommunications techniques, you can begin to utilize more advanced tools to further refine your call-taking skills.

## COMMON TERMS AND PRINCIPLES

Certain words and phrases have come to have commonly understood meanings in progressive systems in our industry. These terms define the methods with which the medical communicator elicits, receives, processes, and prioritizes call information, and with which she or he controls a conversation to better assist the person calling for help.

### Total Acknowledgment

The total acknowledgment is also called an *ack* for short. This is a word or phrase used in three common ways. It is conventionally used to let the caller know that you have heard and understood what she/he has just said. In this case, the call-taker delivers the ack in a neutral tone of voice. While the full ack is most commonly used as just that, an acknowledgment, you can also use it in two more complicated, sophisticated ways. Simply by changing the inflection in your voice and making it more positive, you may use an ack to encourage the caller to continue the conversation in the same direction in which it is heading. By changing the inflection in your voice again to sound more negative, you can use an ack to stop a conversation and redirect it. This may be necessary when the caller is not clearly and concisely providing you with the information you need to prioritize and dispatch the call.

For example: The phone rings, and you answer it.

Call-Taker: "Acme Ambulance, where do you need us?"

Caller: "I live in the Main Street Apartments, you know? They're in the 4800 block of North Main, you know?" (The caller has provided you with the first and most important piece of information needed for dispatch. She is headed in the right general direction, so you want to encourage her to continue. Use a positive, encouraging tone of voice.)

Call-Taker: "Yes, ma'am..."

Caller: "And so this guy, he ran up to my door, you know? And he said to call an ambulance." (Now you need to take charge of the conversation and direct it. You need to know the call-back number and what is wrong. Change your tone of voice. Deliver the ack in a cool, authoritative tone; then ask the questions in a more positive, sympathetic tone.)

Call-Taker: "Okay, ma'am, what is the phone number where you are?"

Caller: "It's 624-9533."

Call-Taker: "And you're in the 4800 block of North Main?"

Caller: "Right." (You now have enough information to pre-alert the unit. You need more specific information about the situation. Make the next ack in a very firm tone of voice, and then resolutely refuse to allow the caller to wander from the subject again.)

Call-Taker: "Okay. What did the man who came to your door say was wrong?"

Caller: "I don't know what's wrong! He just said to call an ambulance!"

Call-Taker: "Tell me *exactly* what the man said when he came to your door."

Caller: "We need an ambulance here now!"

Call-Taker: "Ma'am, tell me *exactly* what the man said when he came to your door."

Caller: "He said some men were fighting in the street, and somebody was hurt!"

This conversation took a grand total of 20 seconds. Although obviously more information is needed for specific prioritization of the call, through skillful use of voice inflection when delivering *acks*, the call-taker has determined the address, telephone number where the caller can be reached, and what the basic problem is.

Some examples of commonly used acks are:

| | |
|---|---|
| Thanks | Yes, sir |
| Got it! | Yes, ma'am |
| Good | Uh-huh |
| Okay | Yeah |

### The "Half-Ack"

The *half-ack* is another method used to acknowledge that you have heard the speaker, and although it does not encourage her/him, it allows the caller to continue in the direction that the conversation is currently headed. The half-ack is accomplished using the same words as the total ack, but is delivered in a softer tone and with a carefully neutral inflection.

### The Comment

At times, a caller will respond to a carefully phrased, very direct question with a statement that has absolutely no relationship at all to the question asked. For example, you ask a woman calling for her husband who is having chest pain, "Where is the pain?" The caller responds with "I think he's dying." This *comment* does you no good; it does not answer your question, and does not add to pertinent call information. Begin again with a strong ack, and then proceed to repetitive persistence. "Ma'am, where is the pain?"

### The Origination

Occasionally while in the process of providing necessary call information, the caller will suddenly identify for you a critical development on the scene. ("Oh, my God, he's got a gun!" is an *origination guaranteed* to get the call-taker's attention.) Whether this is a real crisis or simply a misconception on the part of the caller, the *information flow normally encountered in the call-taking process stops*. For example, a man calls and calmly says, "My partner cut himself on the leg with a chain saw." At this point, normal procedure would be to elicit the call address and call-back number. You say, "All right, sir, what is the address where the patient is now?" The caller suddenly says, "Oh, my God! There is a big stream of blood squirting out of his groin!" You have lost the caller's attention, and his ability to concentrate and respond to your questions is impaired. The life of the patient may or may not also be at risk. You must stop, obtain more information about the crisis, and give instructions. Only then will you be able to resume normal medical interrogation. You must deal with the origination before any further useful communication can occur.

### The Hysteria Threshold

The term *hysteria threshold* was initially coined by Dr. Jeff Clawson, the originator of the process of medical interrogation.[1] Although early use of the term was limited to emergency situations, we now realize that hysteria occurs in many forms, in many different types of situations, and in degrees both large and small. The hysteria threshold is the point at which you can break through another person's hysteria and virtually force them to calm down, provide you with usable information, and follow instructions. Although we most commonly associate classic hysteria with the critical emergency situation, an identical lack of cooperation in lesser degrees is sometimes displayed by the caller in non-emergency cases. Anything that interferes with the information-gathering process completed during the normal call-taking procedure must be dealt with in one way or another. The same techniques used to calm and direct the hysterical emergency caller can be modified or "toned down" and utilized to manage an angry, impatient, or hostile attitude in one who calls for nonemergency service. *Every person on the planet, no matter how frightened, angry, or out of control, has a hysteria threshold; your job is to find it.* The process of reaching the hysteria threshold will continue to elude those communicators who either do not understand how to reach it, or do not believe it exists.

### Repetitive Persistence

Many times, skillful, compassionate manipulation of the call-taker's voice and carefully planned use of acks and half-acks will allow the call-taker to take control of a conversation. When these tools are not effective, try *repetitive persistence*. Repetitive persistence is a fiendishly effective way in which to disarm the hysterical caller.

The technique is very simple. As a call-taker, you should already be in the habit of making your questions short, simple, and easy to follow. When you ask a question and receive in response a comment or an origination, *simply repeat the question*. Repeat it in *exactly* the same tone of voice and use *exactly* the same words you used before. If the caller again replies inappropriately, *ask the question again in exactly the same way*. Do it over and over until the caller responds with the information you need. If you have never used this technique, you will be *amazed* at how well it works.

Occasionally, a slight variation of this technique will be necessary. In the unlikely event that simple repetitive persistence is not successful within a reasonable period of time, you may try changing your tone of voice slightly with each repetition of the question, making the inflection a little more neutral with each repetition. Strive for a completely impersonal monotone.

---

[1] Jeff J. Clawson, M.D. and Kate Boyd Dernocoeur, EMT-P, "Principles of Emergency Medical Dispatch," Brady Publishing, 1988, page 38.

The most common mistake made when practicing repetitive persistence is a lack of attention on the part of the call-taker to the tone and volume level of her/his own voice. *Great care must be taken and a serious effort made not to buy into the emotional reaction of the caller.* Frequently, call-takers who believe they are practicing repetitive persistence are actually allowing themselves to escalate at least as fast and as far as the caller. This escalation can quickly progress to the point where the call-taker and the caller are simply screaming at each other, and absolutely no information exchange is taking place. With each repetition, the call-taker speaks more loudly; each time the question is asked, the tone becomes a little more demanding, impatient, patronizing. Matching the hysteria level of the caller is an avoidable mistake. Make it a habit to listen to yourself frequently on tape; this will help you to identify and modify bad habits as they develop. *Repetitive persistence works. If it's not working for you, you're not doing it right.*

### "Freak" and "Refreak"

The *freak* occurrence takes place when the caller originally recognizes that an emergency exists. She/he becomes hysterical and out of control. When the caller accesses the system and reaches the trained medical communicator, that dispatcher utilizes the standardized calming techniques outlined above to reach the caller's hysteria threshold. The medical communicator helps the caller to regain control, to calm down, and to provide effective communication.

Even after the communicator has gained control of the conversation, the caller in an emergency situation is still at risk of *"refreaking."*[2]

Refreak can be predicted to occur at specific times during the telephone intervention process, and as a result of specific things that happen on the scene of the emergency. Refreak usually occurs when:

- The medical communicator instructs the caller to check the status of the patient by looking at her/him. The caller sees the critical state of her/his friend, loved one, etc., and becomes hysterical again ("Oh, she looks so awful! She looks like she's dead! I don't think she's breathing anymore! Hurry, please hurry!").
- A real or distorted concept of time passed is realized by the caller. The fear pops up that the paramedics aren't coming, and that the caller will have to deal with this situation forever on her/his own.
- The caller follows pre-arrival instructions without result. Americans watch too much television. The average citizen believes that if a person is shot (anywhere), or if a person hits her/his head on the hearth or the coffee table, they die at once. At the opposite end of the spectrum, many people believe, again-

---

[2] National Academy of Emergency Medical Dispatch Certification Course, Medical Priority Consultants, Inc., 1989.

when they perform CPR on a non-breathing, pulseless patient, the patient will be quickly "cured." If that doesn't happen, fear is expressed during the refreak event when the caller says, "Nothing's working!"
- A friend or loved one arrives on the scene. The calm, rational, directed caller who has been following remote intervention directions perfectly suddenly turns into a bowl of Jell-O incapable of doing anything to help the patient. This is a very common, natural, predictable emotional response in a crisis situation.

Refreak can be controlled if the medical communicator simply repeats the original process that enabled to caller to calm down. If a certain series of steps and phrases worked the first time, there is already a behavior pattern set in the caller's mind. Repeat what worked before.

Refreak can happen many times during a single episode of telephone intervention. Use the same techniques to control it each time. Usually it becomes easier to control with each episode.

## ATTITUDE ADJUSTMENT

I have explained that the same emotions and attitudes displayed by an out of control caller for emergency assistance may also be encountered when receiving a nonemergency call. This is important: *When you encounter hostility from the nonemergency caller, it should serve as a warning sign to you. It should not be interpreted or reacted to simply as an irritant, or as a personal attack on you as the call-taker; it should serve to let you know that there may be something wrong somewhere in the service you are providing.* Identify it; then fix it.

## SUMMARY AND REVIEW

1. Define these terms and explain how and why they work:

   total ack          hysteria threshold
   half-ack           repetitive persistence
   comment            freak
   origination        refreak

2. What trap is the easiest for the medical dispatcher to fall into while using the principles of repetitive persistence?

3. What is the most effective tool with which to reach a hysterical caller's hysteria threshold?

4. In what four situations can a caller be predicted to refreak?

# Chapter 10

# THE PSYCHOLOGY OF DEALING WITH THE PERSON IN CRISIS

*"Be not forgetful to entertain strangers, for thereby some have entertained angels unawares."*
— *New Testament, Hebrews, XIII, 2*

## COMPONENTS OF THE HYSTERICAL RESPONSE

In order to effectively learn to elicit necessary information from those who call for your help, first you must reach an understanding of what actually happens when a medical emergency occurs to a member of the general public. Whether or not it is immediately and consciously recognized, either by you as the call-taker or by the person accessing your system, the fact is this: *For every medical emergency there is an equal or greater psychological emergency.* We all live our lives with the illusion that we are secure and in control of events that affect us in major ways. Suddenly, for the caller, that security and that control *do not exist*. Many times, the person who calls you from the scene is calling for the simple reason that she/he is the person present who usually has the answers or can fix a problem. Suddenly, this authority figure for those on the scene has no answers. The vast majority of those who call for our help have little or no medical training.

Try to feel what the caller must be feeling. She/he is having to rely on strangers for help. Most of the general public has no idea who answers the telephone when they call for medical assistance. They do not know what our levels of training or expertise are. They are forced, by circumstances completely beyond their control, to ask for help from an unknown entity. Most have received little or no education about who their medical care providers are, and have no frame of reference to assume confidence in us. *EACH AND EVERY TIME WE RECEIVE AND PROCESS A CALL FOR HELP, WE MUST GIVE THE CALLER*

*CONFIDENCE, COMFORT, AND REASSURANCE; WE MUST MINISTER NOT ONLY TO THE PHYSICAL, MEDICAL NEEDS OF THE PATIENT, BUT TO THE PSYCHOLOGICAL NEEDS OF THE CALLER AS WELL.*

## ATTACK AND COUNTERATTACK

Many times, the fear and loss of control that the caller feels will manifest in hostility toward the call-taker. In the field, you may have experienced hostility and combativeness from a patient who is agitated because she/he is hypoxic and experiencing changes in mentation. When dealing with a hostile caller in the communications center, it is very easy to "buy into" this process emotionally. However, we cannot allow ourselves to do so. The caller's anger is not really directed at you personally; it is simply a component of the psychological emergency that accompanies the medical crisis.

There are four basic components of the human reaction during conflict (see Figure 2.1). *Conflict can be defined as anything that gets in the way of something we want.* When any two or more persons or entities engage in conflict, at least one of the parties involved is perceived as *attacking* the others. An attack can be very direct or extremely subtle; direct attacks are much easier to defend against than those that are made laterally or indirectly.

Any time we perceive an attack by others, we respond in one of two predictable ways. An attack stimulates our recall of basic survival techniques. It is a form of stress, and as such, triggers certain specific reactions. *When we believe ourselves to be under attack, we either counterattack or attempt to escape.* The counterattack, like the initial attack, may be direct or indirect, personal or professional, blatant and crude, or sophisticated and subtle. The other predictable method used to fend off an attack is the *escape*. This is also a component of our basic survival instincts (fright or flight mechanism). There are those who are so accomplished in escape maneuvers that their attackers never even realize that their prey has run away.

A very human response to another person's attempt to escape is the *pursuit*. We live in a society that is competitive by nature; when we perceive a weakness, we pursue and attack again.

In the dispatch setting, callers' hostility and anger must be dealt with in much the same manner as is used when these emotions are encountered in the field. You must depersonalize the experience and assist your callers in regaining control of themselves and of the situation. In most instances, the callers' aggressive behavior will stop as soon as they have received some reassurance from you. It is at this point that they begin to understand that the situation is now under control (if the caller is not calm and in control, then the call-taker *must* be). It is also at this point that the caller becomes most easily guided and most accepting of pre-arrival instructions. You will quickly learn that your conversation with the caller will last a limited time; when you are presented with or can create the opportunity to take control and give the caller real, physical things to do to help the patient, you must do so, calmly and quickly.

## CATEGORIZING OUR CALLERS

Who are the people who call for emergency medical assistance? Approximately half of a system's callers fall into the category of *first-* or *second-party callers*.[1] First-party callers are the persons actually experiencing the problem; they are the patients themselves. Overall, the most beneficial exchange of information takes place with first-party callers. Not only can they give you exact, first-hand information about the problem, but you can give to them instruction, comfort, and reassurance.

Second-party callers are those who are directly involved with the patient. They may have witnessed the event that precipitated the call for help; they may have the patient in sight as they speak to you. They can give you valuable information about the event, history, scene access, and scene hazards. They can also be instructed in pre-arrival actions that may save the patient's life. First- and second-party callers are usually able to give you all the information you need to correctly prioritize the call.

The remaining 50 percent of your calls will come from *third-party callers*.[2] These persons are not in direct contact with the patient (i.e. "I saw a car accident about a mile back on the freeway"). Third-party callers can frequently give only the address, and sometimes a brief description of the problem. However, *it is important that you not assign a caller to the third-party category too quickly*. If the caller is removed from the patient by a relatively short distance (next door, across the street, etc.) because there is no telephone at the encounter address, she/he may be able to return to the scene to obtain more information or instruct those who are in direct contact with the patient to bring the patient to the telephone. When the caller is considerably more removed from the patient ("I saw a traffic accident about two miles east of here"), she or he can be instructed to go back to where the patient is, and at least attempt to minimize the damage.

*Even if the call has already been prioritized and sent up for dispatch, it is important that you stay on the telephone with the caller and at least attempt to give pre-arrival instructions.*

## BUILDING A MENTAL PICTURE

Again, when trying to gain an understanding of the caller and the situation she/he is facing, try to put yourself in the caller's position. From the information you are given, try to picture the physical sur-

---

[1] Clawson and Dernocoeur, EMT-P, "Principles of Emergency Medical Dispatch," p. 35.

[2] Clawson and Dernocoeur, Ibid.

roundings of the patient and the caller. Mentally place yourself in the room with the caller. This caller, like most people, may never before have experienced the need to call for emergency medical help. Picture the caller in the environment from which she/he is calling and trying to handle the specific problem. Now pull the caller out of the picture; substitute a nonmedically trained member of your family or a loved one in the caller's place. The lives of our callers have taken a series of unpredicted turns, and they have no idea how to respond. All of us have, to some degree, been programmed to help those in trouble. When one is faced with a problem that she/he perceives to be critical, the most immediate reaction is to help. If the caller does not know *how* to help, then there is an immediate psychological reaction, accompanied by an actual physical response. As a result of the psychological distress, the caller begins to shake and sweat. She/he may hyperventilate, become nauseated, or actually experience a loss of consciousness.

## SOMEONE ELSE'S SHOES

Several years ago, before enhanced 9-1-1 was in place in my service area, I received a call from a young woman who was absolutely out of her mind with fear. She could *not* stop screaming, and I couldn't understand a word she said. I could hear what sounded like a rational male voice speaking behind her, so I convinced her to hand the phone to her friend. The young man who came on the line was quite calm; he quickly and clearly gave me the information I needed to send the call up for dispatch.

He said that a male friend had attempted suicide at the given address by cutting both his wrists very deeply. The patient had stayed conscious for 10 or 15 minutes while the caller had "tried to stop the bleeding." The patient was breathing, but was now unconscious on the floor of the apartment. When I asked if the bleeding was controlled now, he said, "No; I've been holding pressure on the cuts for at least 10 minutes, and it hasn't stopped yet." I was immediately concerned about the possibility of a major, uncontrolled arterial bleed. I didn't know whether to have the caller repeat the process of applying direct pressure, this time with my direction, or to go for pressure points. Explaining how to find pressure points on a patient with no blood pressure is very difficult to do over the telephone.

About that time, the woman began screaming hysterically again, and I had to raise my voice to be heard. I asked the caller, "Is the blood dark and flowing out in a steady stream, or is it bright red and squirting?"

"I don't know," he answered quietly. "I can't see the cuts that well."

With a clear picture in my head of the last of the patient's blood squirting out onto the floor, I completely lost my patience. "Well," I told him very sternly, "Look at the cuts now! Just bend down there and look!"

"Okay," he said in a quiet, resigned tone of voice. "Hang on a minute."

He was too quiet and too calm. I should have known better.

Three seconds later I heard a faint sighing sound and then a sickening thud. The phone bounced around on the floor, and no one picked it up again until our field crew arrived on the scene. The caller had looked too closely at the blood, and had passed out on top of the patient.

This caller had no medical training; he had no concept of what volume of blood loss can be fatal. He had been applying very delicate pressure with a single square of gauze to each of his friend's wrists (because he didn't want to hurt him), and removing the bandages to look at the wounds every few seconds (to see if it was working). The lacerations were superficial; yet, when the caller continued to see blood trickling from the patient's wrists, he sincerely believed his friend was dying. Both patient and caller were transported to the hospital.

This young man did his best to deal with the crazy woman on the scene, and to follow my instructions. He was completely out of his element, and was extremely nauseated from the time he saw the first drop of blood. Although this call is funny to me now in a sick sort of way, my videotape runs with amplified sound, and the memory of the noise he made when he hit the floor still makes me want to lie down in the road and wait for a bus.

## DEALING WITH THE ELDERLY CALLER

With some callers, particularly the very old or the very young, special considerations are necessary if you are to obtain any usable information. Again, mastering these techniques is simply a matter of putting yourself in the caller's place and treating the caller as you would want to be treated in the same situation.

The key word to remember in successfully addressing the needs of the very elderly caller is *respect*. Some older persons honestly have no idea what to expect when they call for our help. They may clearly remember the days when ambulances were simply funeral home station wagons sent to pick up those who were past needing any help at all. They may interpret your normally successful, assertive, and even aggressive telephone interrogation techniques as simple rudeness. *They may see your rapid-fire questions as an attack; when they do, they have the ability to completely stop the information-gathering process until you have shown them the respect to which they're accustomed.* They frequently view your questions as being evidence of your nosy nature; they honestly believe that the details of the situation are none of your business. They don't understand who we are and what we do.

You don't have time to give these callers a quick history of emergency medical service, or to list the extent of your training and credentials for them. You're not going to be able, in the time you have with the caller, to educate her or him about what progress has been made in the last 20 years in EMS, or what a wonderful system is in place in your service area. Although we in EMS tend to forget this, *it is not the caller's responsibility* to know who we are or what we do for a living. It is, however, *our* responsibility to get the caller the help she or he needs.

How can you accomplish this with an uncooperative caller? Just change your tone of voice. Be sympathetic and, above all, respectful. Say, "Yes, ma'am," and "Yes, sir." Exaggerate the concern in your voice. Treat the caller as you would want your own grandparent treated in the same situation.

## HOW TO TALK TO CHILDREN

Communicating effectively with the very young presents a slightly different problem than that encountered with the very old. While an older person may require respect and the dignity of at least maintaining the illusion that they are in control, the very young frequently want that control taken away from them.

You have been encouraged repeatedly in this text to conduct yourself professionally, to remain neutral, and not to buy into the emotional distress of the caller. In this one instance, throw all that out the window. Children in crisis are accustomed to having older and hopefully wiser adults take control and *help* them in crisis situations. Now, for some reason, their authority figure is either not present, or is incapacitated. This caller needs your emotional involvement, your reassurance, and any comfort you can offer.

Every attempt should be made to stay on the phone with the very young caller. Let your sympathy be heard in your voice. Comfort this child with your voice as you would give her or him a hug if you were physically present on the scene. If the situation on the scene seems to have a grim prognosis, concentrate on minimizing the emotional damage to the caller. Try to find some way to help the child help the patient. *When the call is over, we want this child to know that she or he did everything right.* At the conclusion of your conversation with a child calling for help, always say, "You did a great job. You did everything just right. Thank you for your help."

As a medical professional, you must take great care not to be damaged yourself by interaction with pediatric callers. Dealing with children who are afraid or in pain is as difficult and as draining in the dispatch center as it is in the field. The strain of not being able to physically *be there* for children in trouble takes its toll.

When you "botch" a pediatric call (and you will eventually at least *feel* like you have; we all do, sooner or later), take some steps to prevent yourself from self-destructing over it. Tell someone about the call. Tell them how it made you feel. Recreate the conversation for a friend, colleague, or supervisor. Make a tape recording of the call. Listen to it again and again. After a number of repetitions, you will be able to hear the conversation more cleanly, and with less emotional involvement. Really *hear* what you said to the caller; recognize the comfort and reassurance that you were able to give, even under difficult circumstances. Then outline for yourself what you could have done better, and make the commitment to improve your performance when the situation occurs again.

## HOW IMPORTANT IS YOUR REACTION TO PANIC?

In order for your performance as a system status call-taker to be satisfactory, you *must* learn to tolerate panic, confusion, anger, or other strong emotion on the part of the caller. Why? Because your ability to depersonalize the experience and gain control of the telephone conversation *DIRECTLY IMPACTS PATIENT CARE. Always, always* remember that as medical communicators, utilizing every opportunity to provide excellent patient care is our top priority.

## SUMMARY AND REVIEW

1. What are the two major components of the hysterical response?

2. What four words must you remember about human interactions during crises?

3. Define first-, second-, and third-party callers.

4. What is the key word to remember when dealing with elderly callers?

5. What is the key word to remember when talking with very young callers?

6. What is the most important reason the medical communicator must learn to deal effectively with the panic response?

# Chapter 11

## RECEIVING AND PROCESSING THE CALL FOR ASSISTANCE

*"These are the times that try men's souls."*
— *Thomas Paine, "The American Crisis"*

REVIEW: FIRST CONTACT WITH THE PUBLIC

When you answer any telephone in your communications center, you have under your control what the caller's attitude will ultimately be toward your entire EMS system. The caller's first impression of your system will be a lasting one. *It is vital that each and every telephone call be answered by a calm, controlled, caring medical professional.* Rudeness, discourtesy, or lack of cooperation in any form simply cannot be tolerated.

The SSC must receive and record calls for medical assistance from various sources. This function includes the establishment of effective communication with the person requesting assistance, eliciting of information necessary for the dispatch of an effective response, and the selection of the most appropriate system action in response to each call.

PROVISION OF MEDICAL INFORMATION

The medical communicator is the initial contact with the caller and must be prepared to provide emergency care instructions to callers waiting for the arrival of EMS personnel. These instructions should enable the caller to prevent or reduce further injury to the victim and to do as much as possible under the circumstances to intervene in any life-threatening situation that exists.

The medical dispatcher is also responsible for relaying pertinent medical information to responding units, both for the ultimate benefit of the patient and for the safety of responding personnel.

## TIMELY AND APPROPRIATE ASSIGNMENT OF RESOURCES

Each medical communicator must select and dispatch the necessary vehicles and personnel to the scene of a emergency medical response in the shortest possible time. Each system has its own standards for the maximum allowable seconds for the dispatchers' "chute" times; a tough, but recommended standard is that each communicator be required to consistently dispatch no fewer than 90 percent of emergency responses in 60 seconds or less.

The communicator also functions in coordinating the movements of EMS vehicles en route to the scene, en route to the medical facility or destination, and in returning to service and assignment to a deployment location. This requires that the SSC have up-to-date knowledge of the status of all resources in the service area and the geographic constraints that will affect the medical response. The controller must also have specific medical training and understand the use of rapid reference interrogation and response assignment protocols.

## COORDINATION WITH OTHER PUBLIC SAFETY SERVICES

The SSC must ensure the existence and maintenance of an effective communications link between and among all public safety services (fire, police, helicopter, first responders, etc.) involved in the emergency medical response to facilitate mutual aid and coordination of services such as traffic control, fire suppression, extrication, and rapid transport.

## ELICITING AND RECORDING DISPATCH INFORMATION: ANSWERING THE TELEPHONE

First, always answer the telephone appropriately: "Acme Ambulance, where do you need us?" for emergency lines, and "Acme Ambulance, how may I help you?" for nonemergency lines.

## THE THREE ESSENTIAL ELEMENTS

Before you pick up the telephone, remind yourself of the three critical pieces of information you must have prior to dispatch: *the address, a call-back number, and the nature of the problem.*

Obtain from the caller the exact address or location where the ambulance response is needed. Include:

- The exact address (numbers, street name [spelled if necessary], direction (North Maple) and type (Street, Avenue, Lane, Court, etc.)

- If an exact address is not known, obtain the names of two nearby intersecting streets (Maple and North Main); include direction of travel on highways
- Is the incident location a private residence (house), an apartment, or a business?
- For apartments, obtain the name of the apartment complex, the building number, and the apartment number; or, if applicable, the exact location within the complex (by the pool between buildings 400 and 401 on the north side of the complex)
- For a business, obtain the name of the business, the building or suite number, floor or other incident location identifier, and which entrance to use. If unsure, ask again for *identifiers*: the gate on the side of the building where the logo is, the parking lot without a fence, the corner of the building next to the gas station
- If the caller cannot be specific, have her/him look for and meet the EMS responders

## RECEIVING THE NONEMERGENCY CALL

For nonemergency situations, different yet still specific information is necessary:

- In hospitals, obtain remote building name, if applicable, and room number. For specific departments (X-Ray, Cath Lab, etc.) ask for building name and floor.
- In nursing homes, obtain station or hall designation (station 2, south hall), as well as the room number.
- For scheduled transports, specific additional information is needed:
  - When transporting to a residence, have the caller spell the street name, and ask what city it is in.
  - When transporting to a hospital, ask if the patient is to be transported to the emergency department or other out-patient department, or for direct admission. If being directly admitted, ask if the caller knows the room number to which the patient is scheduled to be admitted.
  - When transporting to a physician's office, ask for the doctor's name, the name of the building (Surgery Associates, Northside Clinic), and the suite or office number.
  - When transporting to an extended care facility, ask for the name of the facility and the address (for example, in any service area there frequently may be several nursing facilities in a "chain," which may have names that are similar.
  - Obtain the caller's full name and telephone number, complete with extension. If your response is delayed, a follow-up call will be required.
  - Ask precisely what the appointment is for. "Special Studies" or

tests that may be critical to patient care (heart caths, CT scans) indicate special dispatch considerations.
- Ask what time the patient will be ready, or what time the appointment is scheduled.
- Consider negotiating a pick-up time. If the transport is not for a scheduled appointment and the patient is ready now, check the current call load, number of nonemergency transfers already awaiting dispatch, and the current system level. You may wish to tell the caller, "We can pick Mrs. Jones up within 45 minutes (or other time frame, depending on the status of the system)." This practice can facilitate effective on-line system management, and can improve customer satisfaction by giving the caller a realistic expectation of when the transport ambulance will arrive. Don't accept a scheduled pick-up time if you know you will be late; attempt to renegotiate the pick-up time. When practicing this type of scheduling, be sure to "time-stamp" each event, so that later you will have a clear record of what time the call was received, what pick-up time was arranged, and what time the unit actually arrived.
- For every type of request for assistance, obtain from the caller the telephone number, including extension, where the caller and/or the patient can be reached.
- Obtain from the caller the nature of the problem to determine the presumptive patient condition code.
- Follow medical prioritization protocols *exactly, every time* to correctly prioritize the call and dispatch appropriate units.

## KEY QUESTIONS

The most critical call information will be obtained by asking and noting the answers to the following *key questions*. These questions must be asked and answered during any request for medical assistance:

- *Where?* What is the exact address of the patient/incident? Where did the incident occur? Where should the responding units be sent? How can the responding units get there quickly and efficiently?
- *What* is the *telephone number* where the caller is? What is the telephone number where the patient is?
- *What's wrong there?* What kind of problems is the patient having? What has happened? What type of response is needed (use protocols)?
- *Who* is calling? Is the caller from the general public or from a public safety agency? What agency? *Who* is the person needing help? Is the caller with the patient? Does the caller have only third-party information?
- *How old* is the patient?
- Is the patient *awake and talking*?

- Is the patient *breathing* okay?
- *When* did the incident occur? How long has it been going on? In cases of violent crime (shootings, stabbings, assaults), is the person who did it still there?

Answers to these key questions provide the information necessary to adequately establish the priority of medical response. Other key questions asked for medical cases as opposed to traumatic situations will differ slightly.

*Questioning during medical interrogation must be kept short.* Ask one question at a time, *and wait for the caller to answer.* Rapid-fire questioning can be very confusing to the caller.

In *medical* cases, key questions are usually based on *symptoms*.

- Is the patient *awake and talking*?
- Is the patient *breathing* okay?
- *How old* is the patient?
- Is the patient having any *chest pain*?

The caller is usually with the patient and/or is familiar with the patient and her/his problems. *Always refer to prioritization protocols for the specific condition indicated.*

In *traumatic* incidents, key questions are generally based on the *type of incident or the mechanism of injury* rather than specific symptoms, since the caller is frequently a third-party observer and is not with the patient.

- Is the patient *awake and talking*?
- Is the patient *breathing* okay?
- *How old* is the patient?
- *Where* is she/he shot? *How far* did she/he fall? *Where* is she/he injured?

The answers to questions in the fourth category above will identify prioritization differences for different traumatic situations. *Always refer to prioritization protocols for the specific condition indicated.*

## THIRD-PARTY LIMITATIONS

This system of utilizing medical interrogation via key questions is based on the idealistic concept that all the information asked for by the call-taker is available from the caller. Obviously, this is not always the case. The intelligent interrogator must occasionally modify her/his questioning as appropriate. *When there is not enough information available to reduce the response level according to the protocols, it is advisable to dispatch the maximum response for that condition.*

## CONTINUING THE PROCESS

Follow the prioritization protocols *exactly, every time* for the specific patient condition indicated. Record all the pertinent information, either in a CAD system via the call entry screen or manual dispatch card. Make a written note of any special identifiers, patient information, or access instructions into the remarks field on the call entry screen. Remember that information contained in the remarks section of any response documentation is a legal document subject to subpoena. "Meet the idiot at the pay phone" is not acceptable. If the permanent record goes to court, the medical communicators involved also have to go to court, and explain their actions. *Don't humiliate yourself or your colleagues in the system in public.*

*Record all information as accurately and as fully as possible. Do not rely on your memory; record everything.*

Prioritization of information should be completed quickly. As soon as an element is identified that establishes the priority at which the call must be dispatched, *enter the call (if using a CAD system), send up the call for dispatch (if more than one communicator is on duty), pre-alert the appropriate unit, or dispatch the response.* Once an answer to your questions has been given which dictates the level of the response, dispatch *must not* be delayed while additional information is gathered to clarify the situation on the scene or direct the call-taker in providing pre-arrival instructions.

As you enter the call and send it up for dispatch, reassure the caller that help is on the way, and explain what you are doing. For example, "Ma'am, I've sent the call up by computer (every person who owns a television set will form an immediate mental picture from this phrase, and will take comfort from it), and the paramedics are on the way. I am also a paramedic. *Now, let me tell you what to do until the others arrive.*"

When the prioritization process is complete and the call has been entered and sent up for dispatch, give remote intervention instructions as necessary. *Follow the medically approved protocols.* The SSC should also obtain pertinent medical history and/or special information about the scene, and relay that information to responding units. She/he must relay information

between various units and agencies. If a fire or police response is indicated, the SSC must make sure the responding agency has been notified and has all pertinent information.

## OFFERING A DIFFERENT KIND OF HELP

There will be times when the caller has done all she/he can do, or when she/he is unable to get to the patient to give any aid. There will also be situations where the caller is too young, too elderly, or too infirm to be able to follow and perform remote intervention instructions. In these cases, the call-taker can at least assist in keeping the caller calm, by suggesting such activities as:

- Gathering the patient's medications
- Unlocking the door
- Turning on the porch lights, etc.
- Anything else that will help to get the caller's mind off what she/he cannot do and get her/him to do something positive

## FOLLOWING THROUGH

When the call has been dispatched, it is the shared responsibility of the call-taker and the radio operator to follow the progression of the call, monitoring status changes closely. Check to make sure all changes in unit status are received, acknowledged, and logged. Watch for delays in response times.

Use the CAD system if one is available. If, in the early phases of your training, you are concentrating so hard on entering information correctly into the CAD that you are missing some of what's being said to you, you may write the information down and then enter it. If you are having this problem, additional training and drilling in typing skills will probably be required. The goal for this type of training should be for each communicator to have the typing skills and speed to be able to enter call information directly into the CAD as the caller gives it.

## SUMMARY AND REVIEW

1. What should you say when you answer an emergency telephone line?

2. How should you answer a nonemergency telephone line?

3. What are the three information items essential for dispatch?

4. Which two items from problem 3 could you conceivably do without if you had to?

5. Generally speaking, do you need more information to send an emergency response or a nonemergency response? Why?

6. What are some of the standard key questions for medical patients? For trauma patients? Why is there such a difference?

7. What percentage of those who call for help are third-party callers?

8. If circumstances prevent the successful use of remote intervention techniques, is there anything else you can do to help the caller?

# Chapter 12

# RADIO COMMUNICATIONS

*"Blessed is the man who, having nothing to say,
abstains from giving us wordy evidence of the fact."*
— George Eliot, "Theophrastus Such"

## WHO ARE YOU AND WHY ARE YOU HERE?

Just as your telephone demeanor will define your system's image with the general public, your department's radio attitude and procedures will largely determine the nature of your relationship with your system's field care-givers. Granted, you can do this job without full, voluntary cooperation from field personnel; any command or administrative staff can write into policy both behavioral criteria for field personnel and standardized disciplinary procedures to be rigidly followed when those criteria are not met. However, that's not the point. It is infinitely easier to achieve excellence when all parties adopt a supportive, cooperative role rather than an adversarial one. We are all players on the same team; we all desire the same positive end result. Being at war with other agencies, departments, or divisions is in direct conflict with the challenge accepted by field and communications personnel alike: to provide a constant, vigilant attempt to decrease the incidence of death, reduce human suffering, and protect the dignity of others.

Take a good look at both the general departmental attitude and the specific policies and procedures in place for your communications personnel. While today's medical dispatchers play a very active role in patient care, our primary function remains the same: to provide information, resources, and support for those who deliver hands-on patient care in the field setting. By doing your job well, you help your system's field personnel to do the same. This improves the general quality of care administered to the citizens in your service area. *Every communications policy and procedure and every radio transmission you make should reflect this motivation.*

## ANOTHER CHANGE IN PERSPECTIVE

If you drew a time line that reflected the elapsed years between the present time and the period when emergency pre-hospital care was first provided by ambulance personnel, mobile radios would actually appear as an afterthought. Emergency services existed for a number of years before mobile radio equipment was considered to be as critical as it is today. While the provision of the radio communications link to ambulance personnel was once employed largely as a novelty, functional radio equipment is now considered to be a critical piece of apparatus. In the majority of response systems today, units without operational radios are regarded as out of service and unavailable. What if the crew has a motor vehicle accident? Without a radio, they can't even tell you they're in trouble. What if they're being attacked, or find themselves caught in an otherwise violent situation? Without a functional radio, they can't call for help. What if you need to relay to them important information relevant to a response? Without the mobile radio, field personnel are condemned to response situations where the initial information received about any call must be considered accurate. Without mobile radio communication, there is no link between people who need information and those who have it. The very fact that this radio connection is considered such a vital part of response readiness should establish in each medical dispatcher's mind the importance of any decision that affects the nature of radio communication.

## RADIO CODES AND SIGNALS OR PLAIN ENGLISH?

In any emergency response system, one of the first issues to be addressed is the format in which your radio communications will be conducted. Do the employees of your system currently transmit call-related information in plain English, or through a series of radio codes and signals? If codes and signals are used, do you know why?

Wait a minute, now; I'm not asking for the reasons that the use of codes was first implemented. I'm talking about now, today. What purpose do the signals serve in your system today? Do they fulfill the purpose for which they were originally intended? *Do they serve any purpose at all? Do your system's communicators have any idea why they're doing things the way they do?*

In most systems, the practice of transmitting coded information rather than plain English was implemented for several reasons. At first glance, they were good reasons; however, whether they weren't completely thought through or whether times have changed, in most areas the process is simply not working. It is not achieving its original goal.

Administrators and commanders in systems that utilize codes and signals exclusively will tell you that the practice is beneficial in many ways: communication is faster and cleaner. It is more efficient. Radio codes and signals protect confidential information and help to maintain the privacy of the patient.

In the real world, the practice of coding response-related information usually achieves none of the goals listed above. The information exchange is not faster if numbers must be repeated. It is not cleaner if the data is first transmitted in code, and then must be explained or clarified over the radio channel. Learning a complex system of signals and codes lengthens the training time for any new employee, and public safety organizations within the same service area often use the same numbers to mean completely different things. By their nature, call-related radio transmissions contain many numbers: street addresses, map references, incident or run numbers, and so on. When you add more numbers to the process, you increase the risk for error. Number identifiers transmitted over a radio channel are easily misunderstood, and may be transposed.

If your goal is to protect the privacy of your patient and the confidentiality of patient-related information, give it up. In every service area, lists of radio frequency assignments are available. Private citizens with scanners (some of which are more sophisticated and expensive than your dispatching equipment) constantly monitor the transmissions of fire, police, and EMS services. Anyone who wants to know what your codes and signals mean will access that information in very short order. In some systems, amateur radio enthusiasts have a clearer understanding of the radio signals in use than do the employees of the system itself. However, if clear English is exclusively used, then all information, even that which is not response related or is of a confidential or sensitive nature, is available to anyone who is affluent enough to purchase a scanner, and intelligent enough to program it. What's the answer?

The most practical, workable solution to this problem seems to be found in compromise between the two extremes. Response and transport information can be relayed in plain, easily understood English. A limited number of codes or signals may be used to identify elements or events important only from an internal system perspective. For example, changes in unit status such as crews checking out for meal breaks, available for emergency response only, or approaching their designated shift end may be broadcast in abbreviated, easily understood codes or signals. In this instance, coded information can actually reduce confusion and limit the amount of air time expended on nonemergency radio transmissions.

## RADIO OPERATIONS: A PROCEDURAL OVERVIEW

The medical communicator occupying the position of radio operator can and does literally set the tone for the entire work force and service area simply by the inflection in her/his voice. The radio operator must at all times maintain professional radio conduct. She/he must maintain a pleasant, even, well-modulated, nonirritating tone of voice. She/he must not convey "attitude" on the radio.

When a field crewperson transmits inappropriately over a radio channel, the radio operator simply must not respond in kind, but must maintain professionalism while transmitting. If there is a problem with a crew's conduct on the radio channel, the radio operator should request that the incident be resolved through the established chain of command. Document the occurrence of the inappropriate behavior, pull audio recordings of the transmission, and notify a field operations supervisor, but do not respond to the event by displaying inappropriate attitude of your own. Don't act stupid in public.

Inappropriate radio conduct by a communicator should be cause for disciplinary action in any system and should not be tolerated. You are supposed to be setting a professional example.

The radio operator must at all times transmit in a calm, collected manner. *When stress is evident in a controller's voice, the stress level in the field escalates accordingly.* Higher stress in the field can actually impair the safety of the field crews and can negatively impact the delivery of excellent patient care.

The radio operator's position may be considered a temporary, rotating supervisory position. Only one communicator should be designated as radio operator at one time. Except in isolated cases of communications center overload, any radio transmissions should be made by the designated radio operator, and not by the medical dispatchers occupying call-taking positions. Transmissions by multiple SSCs can be both confusing and irritating to field personnel.

Any decisions concerning changes in the status of the system should be cleared by the controller occupying the radio operator's position. Try to avoid any action or transmission that will sound rushed, hurried, or stressed.

For both medical and legal reasons, the radio operator should clearly state the time on the main dispatch channel **each** time a unit verbally transmits a status change.

## PRE-ALERTING APPROPRIATE FIELD UNITS

Alerting the appropriate field unit to an upcoming response *before the actual dispatch* can significantly reduce the practical total response time for any call. Especially when the call-taker has difficulty obtaining pertinent medical and scene information, the practice of pre-alerting the response can give field personnel up to a 4- or 5-minute "head start."

How is pre-alerting achieved? The communicator acting as radio operator "keys in" on each emergency line as it is answered by a call-taker. The radio operator listens long enough to identify:

- The address and/or location where help is needed, and
- The nature of the problem as initially stated by the caller

When these two pieces of information have been given, the radio operator "unkeys" from the phone line, and identifies and pre-alerts the closest appropriate unit. With very few exceptions, the radio operator should be able to place the general area of the incident location *as soon as a street name or telephone exchange is identified*. Extensive geographic knowledge of the service area is a required job skill for the professional medical dispatcher. One or two *quick* attempts may be made to contact a unit by radio, if the radio operator believes the crew to be mobile in their unit. Otherwise, the appropriate unit should be paged or otherwise "toned out" and pre-alerted to respond.

What verbiage should be used to accomplish a pre-alert? Some suggestions are:

"Medic 21, pending priority 2, 4500 North Main, map reference 45 N-Nora." or

"Medic 21, pending priority 2, 4500 North Main, district 7."

"Medic 21, clear for a call!" is acceptable, I suppose; however, this type of transmission sounds rushed and incompetent. The stress in your voice causes stress levels for field personnel to escalate proportionally. *If you have enough information to know which unit to send, you have enough information to correctly phrase the pre-alert.* Formats and styles for pre-alerting must be consistent between dispatchers, and must be agreed upon by the entire communications department. Acceptable formats are acceptable because they provide responding crews with concise, practical, *usable information*.

## DISPATCHING THE RESPONSE

When the call-taker has triaged the call information and reached a decision for response prioritization, the radio operator assigns a specific unit to the response and dispatches the call. This process may involve the use of a CAD system or manual dispatch cards.

Suggested verbiage to be used when dispatching a call is:

"Medic 21, priority 2, injured person; 4500 North Main, 4-5-0-0 North Main, map reference 45 N-Nora, cross street Elm Avenue, incident number 1234, one-two-three-four, responding at 0745."

The format for dispatching nonemergency calls should be virtually identical to that above. When dispatching any unit, include specific information as discussed (apartment complex name, building number, apartment number, name of business, etc.).

When the unit has been dispatched to respond, it becomes the shared responsibility of the call-taker and the radio operator to monitor radio traffic for unit status changes. If your system uses manual dispatch cards, all dispatchers on duty should make sure that status changes are appropriately time-stamped. If you are utilizing a CAD system with mobile data terminals, all communicators should monitor unit status screens to make sure each data signal is received, acknowledged, and logged at the same time as the voice transmission.

## ACKNOWLEDGING UNIT TRANSMISSIONS

When a unit verbally transmits a status change, the radio operator should acknowledge the information reported and *state the time, every time*. For example:

| | |
|---|---|
| Unit: | "Medic 21 on scene." |
| SSC: | "Medic 21 on scene, 0748." |
| | or |
| Unit: | "Medic 42 responding." |
| SSC: | "Medic 42 responding, 0752." |

## MAKING POST MOVE-UPS

As soon as a unit has been pre-alerted for a response, the radio operator must adjust the coverage of the service area as appropriate. *The unit deployment plan should be followed, and post move-ups should be made within 15 seconds of any pre-alert or dispatch. In the event that pre-alerting was not possible, the post move-up should be made within 15 seconds of the dispatch that altered coverage.* Only by making post move-ups quickly can you avoid extended response times in the affected parts of your service area.

For as long as the principles of system status management have been utilized to improve response times and increase system efficiency, spirited discussions have taken place concerning the method used when adjusting for changing unit deployment demands. For a time, we all thought that moving units "chain-style" provided more complete unit availability to all parts of the response area. Then we were told that the resulting work load for field personnel nationwide was too intense and must be decreased. At that point, some system administrators decreed that only one unit should be moved when coverage demands changed; we would play the odds and hope that we didn't receive a critical call in an area where no ambulances were located.

Today, as we progress in utilizing the experience and knowledge gained in our own systems and in those of others, most system status managers recognize that an inordinately high number of post move-ups are frequently generated by another source. At low system levels, any plan for unit deployment can actually be *too precise*. Deployment programs cannot be designed solely on the basis of statistical information. In larger service areas, the geographic component must receive careful consideration as well. This alone will significantly decrease the number of post move-ups in any given hour.

The number of post changes made by field crews can further be reduced by agreeing to (what a surprise) compromise on the methods of unit movement employed. At or below a designated cutoff level (which should reflect the historical number of emergency responses made during the hour), or when coverage is compromised to a large or very active portion of the service area, chain-style movements are indicated. When the system is solidly above cutoff level, and only low-volume areas are left to be covered, then one unit can be moved with a high degree of success.

## SUMMARY AND REVIEW

1. What are the two primary roles of the medical communicator?

2. Do you see yourself as providing support for your system's field crews?

3. Does your system use plain English, radio codes and signals, or a combination of the two? Do you know why?

4. What FCC rules and regulations address the issue of professionalism when broadcasting over a radio channel?

5. What communication method is used in your system to provide direct-voice contact between hospital personnel and field care-givers?

6. In your system, can those communications channels be secured for privacy?

7. Do medical dispatchers in your system aggressively pre-alert field units to upcoming responses? If not, why not?

8. Does your department have in place a standardized and approved format for pre-alerting and dispatching field units?

9. Are the principles of system status management in use in your service area? Which method (one unit or "chain-style" movement) is used to direct unit movement from one posting location to another? Why?

Chapter **13**

# MEDICOLEGAL ISSUES IN EMERGENCY MEDICAL DISPATCHING

*"I am innocent of any wrongdoing . . . I am the daughter of a freedom fighter . . . That man bullied me . . . Besides, I cannot go to prison. American prisons are full of lesbians."*
— *Zsa Zsa Gabor to the press shortly before her conviction for assault on a police officer*

## OVERVIEW: WELCOME TO THE REAL WORLD

If you are to have any logical understanding of or any realistic expectations about the legal system in this country and your potential involvement with it, there are three basic principles that you must understand:

*First*, that the law has absolutely nothing to do with right or wrong; it is simply *the law*.

*Second*, that anyone can sue anyone else in civil court, anytime, anywhere, and for any reason, *and win*. No one is protected from civil litigation.

*Third*, that, no matter how clearly and precisely a law, statute, or judicial opinion is written, *the interpretation of that writing is subject to change*. These changes occur regularly and in phases. Interpretation of the law is never static. Trends are established, usually reflecting either largely liberal or conservative views, but they always change again. That's why they call them trends.

The focus of litigation relating to emergency medical service has changed in recent years. During the early phase of EMS as an industry, field care was the principal target for legal action; at the present time, the most publicized lawsuits in EMS involve the dispatch function. The focus is on *you* now; the best way for you to protect yourself

## COMMON MISTAKES: DANGER ZONES FOR LITIGATION

*"The American people never carry an umbrella.
They prepare to walk in eternal sunshine."*
— *Alfred E. Smith, speech*

To be forewarned is to be forearmed. What are the most common factors identified in medical dispatch lawsuits? They are:

- Failure to verify information, usually location and callback number
- Failure to send an ambulance (there are at least three major, big-money lawsuits involving this factor pending now)
- A significantly delayed response, usually identified as between 38 and 90 minutes
- Shift change miscommunications. These types of communications errors are common to the field of medical care (rushed and/or incomplete shift reports, missing information, failure to report information); because of two widely publicized cases, this type of error is very much in the mind of the public
- Multiple calls for help: more than one call *in any situation* is *always* a bad sign
- No protocols in place; "re-inventing the wheel" each time the phone rings
- Protocols in place, but not used ("We're smarter than the protocols")
- Failure to provide remote intervention directions; now that the delivery of these instructions is the national standard, the potential for liability exists if they are not given
- Requesting to speak to the patient (when this is asked to prove the caller wrong, not to verify or clarify from a positive perspective)
- Improper identification or management of "hyperventilation": misunderstanding the "rules" for making this determination, not sending an ambulance because this is perceived as a "minor" problem, or inappropriate phone treatment (breathing into a paper bag).[1] *Heads up. Never, never, never, as long as you are employed as a medical communicator, tell anyone under any circumstances to breathe into a paper bag. There is absolutely no way to determine over the telephone whether rapid breathing is due to uncomplicated acute hyperventilation syndrome or a more serious medical or metabolical problem. If the underlying problem is something other than simple hyperventilation syndrome, breath-*

---

[1] Medical Priority Consultants, Inc., 1989.

*ing into a paper bag can critically damage or kill your patient.* If you don't understand this, dig out your textbooks and review the presentation signs of respiratory compromise in various medical and metabolic disorders. If you don't believe it, research the cases currently in litigation nationwide.

- An argumentative and/or nonempathetic attitude: logical or not, right or wrong, fair or unfair, the way this works out is that "both good doctors and bad doctors get sued, but nice doctors don't." [2]

## IMPORTANT LEGAL TERMS AND CONCEPTS AS THEY APPLY TO MEDICAL DISPATCHERS

*"Ignorance of the law excuses no man: not that all men know the law, but because 'tis an excuse every man will plead, and no man can tell how to confute him."*
— *John Selden, "Table-Talk"*

### Duty

When you agree to perform as a care-giver in an EMS provider system, you assume responsibility to provide a certain level of care. *The medical communicator is now included in the category of "caregiver."* Your duties will be determined initially by national and local standards; however, changing social conditions lead constantly to the recognition of new duties. No better general statement can be made than that the courts will find a duty where, in general, reasonable men would recognize it and agree that it exists.[3]

### Negligence

As our industry becomes more sophisticated and our practices better grounded, we naturally (and in most cases, eagerly) assume more responsibility for providing increasingly advanced levels of care. As responsibility increases, the potential for liability increases. The recognition and definition of "duty" as an abstract concept are pivotal in reaching a finding of negligence.

There are four basic elements that traditionally have been necessary to prove negligence:

*First*, that the defendant had a duty to act;
*Second*, that duty was breached, either by acts of commission or omission;
*Third*, that an injury of some kind resulted from that breach of duty;

---

[2] Medical Priority Consultants, ibid.
[3] Clawson and Dernocoeur, EMT-P, "Principles of Emergency Medical Dispatch," p. 205. Citing W. Page Keeton, ed., *Prosser and Keeton on the Law of Torts,* 5th ed. (St. Paul, Minn.: West Publishing Co., 1984), p. 359.

*Fourth*, there must be clear causation, meaning that the cause and effect relationship of the agency's duty to act is clearly related to the injury sustained.[4]

Whereas in traditional theory, the burden of proof rests with that party making the complaint (the plaintiff), it is safe to predict that in actual civil case law, a new trend will soon be established. Even when criminal charges cannot be substantiated, outrageously large sums are often awarded in civil judgments. *The Tort of Outrage* is one mechanism by which all the traditional assumptions about burden of proof may be negated. Basically, the Tort of Outrage allows that a judgment may be found for the plaintiff even when the four elements listed above cannot be met, provided the behavior or attitude of the defendant is established as "outrageous."[5] What this translates into is that four precise and traditional factors have to be established and proven, and those are the rules, and they never change, and this will protect you, *unless you are obnoxious by someone else's standards, which standards will change with local and national trends, and which standards, in any case, will not be established or provided to you until the action goes to trial.*

The Prudent Action Rule

This guideline for governing the behavior of the employee in emergency service is widely used in other industries as well. Basically, this means that you, under a given set of circumstances, must take the same action that any prudent person, trained to your level of expertise and presented with the same set of circumstances, would take.

The Emergency Rule

Hypothetical interpretations of this rule tend to lead the caregiver, in this case the medical dispatcher, to assume that a degree of protection lies in the theory behind the traditional emergency rule. *This tradition states that a person functioning in an emergency situation cannot be held to the same performance level and/or the same expectations of conduct as a person who is not functioning in a state of emergency.* The current presumptive interpretation of this rule as it applies to EMS providers will lead the medical communicator to assume that, if call volume and work activity are high, she/he is not expected to perform as well as when activity levels are low. *I believe this is a misleading interpretation that will eventually, although perhaps indirectly, lead to disastrous results in EMS litigation.*

If the "overload" or "emergency" situation occurs with any frequency or regularity, it becomes the responsibility of the communicator to identify the problem to her/his supervisor; then, it becomes the

---

[4] Clawson and Dernocoeur, ibid., pp. 205-06.
[5] Medical Priority Consultants, ibid.

responsibility of the administrator of that department, division, or agency to provide better planning, preparation, and support, so that the *quality* of service continues at a consistent level even when personnel in the dispatch center are very busy. Information from EMS systems nationwide will only serve to establish that this standard of obligation and this delineation of responsibility already exist.

A frequently asked question is, "If remote intervention directions are provided to one caller in a critical situation (i.e., life-saving CPR instructions), but are not given to another caller experiencing the same critical situation because call volume is so high that there is simply not enough time to do so, will the medical dispatcher be liable for not providing the instructions in the second case?" I do not believe that this is a practical example of where the greatest danger lies in interpreting the emergency rule. In this case, it is very possible that the court system would not have unreasonable expectations of the abilities of the dispatcher. *What I fear is that the medical communicator will adopt the interpretation of the emergency rule as a general, frequent, catch-all excuse for substandard performance, and that she/he will develop a false sense of security because of it.* When it can be statistically proven that an overload situation did exist, the communicator will in all probability not be held liable for failure to provide complete remote intervention directions to every caller during the period of the overload. *The element of predictability will figure prominently in any interpretation of the emergency rule as it applies to EMD.* When this excuse is unprovable (not documented, and with no data to back up the claim), the medical dispatcher will eventually be left without any viable defense.

### Foreseeability

When applied to our specific situation, this concept basically establishes a precedent for the protection of the medical communicator. It presupposes that if "bad," incorrect, or incomplete information is given by the caller, the system status controller will not be held liable for dispatching errors. Since the dispatcher could not foresee the problem, she/he made the best decision possible under the circumstances. Actual court findings pertaining to this concept will, in all probability, be dependent on current interpretations of other terms in this section, that is, the prudent action rule, the emergency rule, special relationships, detrimental reliance, and so on.

### Deviation from Protocols

*"I am not arguing with you — I am telling you."*
   — *J. McN. Whistler, "The Gentle Art of Making Enemies"*

In a word, *don't.*

Figures compiled in 1989 by Medical Priority Consultants, Inc., indicate that, in surveys of the 200 largest EMS systems nationwide, 61 percent (usually the most widely known, top providers with the best reputations for providing high-quality patient care) had standardized, medically approved dispatching protocols in place.[6] *Figure it out. Sixty-one percent is more than half. That in itself establishes a national standard of care.* Not following in-place protocols will get you in just as much trouble as if the system had never established the protocols at all. Ad-libbing is not acceptable. *Juries are traditionally unsympathetic to those who fail to follow established protocols.*

### Special Relationships

The definition of the term *special relationship* is another that will probably change repeatedly with the interpretations delivered in different cases. Basically, it refers to *promises* made by the *provider* (whether *specifically stated or implied*), and *beliefs* held by the *plaintiff (whether or not the provider took direct action to establish or encourage those beliefs).*[7] A special relationship exists any time there is a contract in place between a provider and the communities it serves. A special relationship also exists in any geographic area where the 9-1-1 emergency notification system is in place. Public relations efforts and advertising by the provider, local news stories, national news exposure, articles in trade magazines, or anything else that, directly or indirectly, leads the public to hold particular expectations, whether clearly stated or implied, all contribute to and can be used to establish the existence of a special relationship.

### Detrimental Reliance

The term *detrimental reliance*[8] refers to those situations where the plaintiff charges that she/he relied on the system, the providing agency, the department, or the individual dispatcher, usually due to the expectations resulting from a special relationship, to the ultimate detriment of the patient.

## FUTURE SHOCK

In summary, while this area of litigation is relatively new and untried, findings on certain issues and in certain areas are already predisposed to move in certain directions. Some attitudes have already been established. Charges revolving around remote intervention directions will involve errors of omission rather than commission. The practice of dispatch prioritization will remain in place as a national standard. The communications training programs of EMS providers will continue to draw fire; standards for training will improve, and will have to be proven again and again.

The value of national certification for medical communicators will be clearly, finally, and permanently established.

---

[6] Medical Priority Consultants, ibid.
[7] Medical Priority Consultants, ibid.
[8] Medical Priority Consultants, ibid.

You can safely anticipate reading about future lawsuits charging that an emergency response was made when it was not medically warranted by the patient's condition. Current figures indicate that over 70,000 traffic accidents, 35,000 injuries, and 700 deaths may occur each year related to emergency medical vehicle responses.[9]

Sounds pretty shaky, huh? Are you scared to death? Are you afraid to answer the telephone? Well, don't be. How can you protect yourself from exposure to litigation? Follow the guidelines contained in this text; consult with your system's legal counsel. Avoid the known danger zones. Demand administrative support, and then help to establish and maintain a good, comprehensive training program. Respect the function of medical control. Develop accurate record-keeping skills. Participate in a functional risk management program. Inform your supervisor of errors and unusual incidents; in turn, you have the right to insist that your supervisor keep you informed of any changes that will affect your ability to perform your job. Master the art of working as a team member. Actively participate in an agressive quality assurance and quality improvement program. Set high standards for yourself and your department, and *always keep the highest quality patient care your top priority*.

## SUMMARY AND REVIEW

1. What are the three things every medical communicator should know about the American legal system?

2. Name ten types of errors committed by medical dispatchers which most frequently result in litigation.

3. Define and explain the following terms and concepts as they apply to medical dispatching:

- duty
- prudent action
- foreseeability
- special relationships
- negligence
- the emergency rule
- deviation from protocols
- detrimental reliance

4. What danger exists if telephone triage is not correctly practiced, an emergency response is dispatched when no medical need exists, and an injury accident results?

5. Can a state of communications center overload be proven?

6. What is the probable extent of your legal liability if you triage a response incorrectly as the result of receiving incorrect information?

7. What future legal trends in emergency medical litigation can safely be predicted?

---

[9] Scott A. Hauert, Lecture: "Medicolegal Aspects of EMS," National Academy of Emergency Medical Dispatch Certification Course, Orlando, Florida, 1989, based on unpublished statistical study.

# Chapter 14

# DOCUMENTATION AND REPORTING TECHNIQUES

*"If it ain't on paper, you ain't got a bitch."*
— *Jack Stout during lecture on effective documentation,
Advanced System Status Management Seminar,
Fourth Party, Inc., Miami, Florida, 1989*

## A CHANGE IN FOCUS

As the duties and responsibilities of the medical dispatcher have changed over the years, the nature and volume of required documentation have also changed. While the role of the dispatcher was subject to linear definition, documentation in the communications center was limited in scope and difficulty. Reporting was frequently in the form a simple log of calls run during any 24-hour period.

The job duties of the medical communicator or system status controller now exist on multiple levels. In different systems, the responsibilities of dispatchers or controllers can include calculation of unit hour demand requirements, scheduling, compliance reporting, the compilation of statistics, and the gathering of information used to facilitate planning for future system needs.

## THE INCREASED NEED FOR DOCUMENTATION

The importance of complete and accurate documentation cannot be too strongly or too frequently stressed. Good documentation will help you to remember a particular incident several years and tens of thousands of calls later. It will protect both you and your system in cases of litigation. It will establish the facts and make clear exactly what did and did not take place. It will also enable you, your department, your company or employer, and the industry as a whole to explain, justify, and defend your actions in any given situation. Documentation allows us to supply figures that prove our compliance with contractual requirements and to justify budget needs to our customers and governing agencies. Accurate, complete, and valid reporting enables us to identify and track factors that impact our performance as a system and as an industry, and to improve patient care by improving our services.

## PRACTICAL TECHNIQUES AND APPLICATIONS

Surprisingly little has been written about the need for complete and accurate documentation in emergency medical service. A minimum of practical, usable information is provided in most emergency medical textbooks; any direction that is available pertains almost exclusively to the reporting of situations encountered during the administration of field care.

The need for reliable reporting in the medical communications center has always existed. In recent years, as the focus of attention for the media and civil litigators has shifted from field care to communications, the necessity of excellent recordkeeping in the dispatch center has become increasingly evident.

## AUDIO RECORDINGS AS DOCUMENTATION

From the field perspective, documentation is almost exclusively written; communications center reporting can be accomplished through use of an additional method. Audio recordings are now commonly used to show a series of actions or a sequence of events. The need for 24-hour audio recording of any communications center's telephone lines, radio channels, and radio-relayed patient reports is now universally recognized. Audio tapes are also frequently used to help with field medical audits, call and chart reviews, and the training and retraining of both field personnel and medical communicators. The long-term protection gained by having access to round-the-clock audio recordings more than compensates for the initial expense of setting up such a recording system. At this stage in the development of our industry, we must not only consistently complete our job duties to meet or exceed a high performance standard, *we must be able to prove on demand that we did so.*

## TIME STAMPING STATUS CHANGES AND IMPORTANT EVENTS

The availability of equipment resources to the workers in each medical response system directly reflects the accessibility of financial resources available to that system, agency, or service area. It's unfortunate, but it's also a fact of life. (This is one of many reasons to contribute at every opportunity to the financial well-being of the company or service that employs you.) Some EMS services utilize sophisticated computer-assisted dispatch (CAD) systems that automatically record the time at which each event or status change occurs. At the other end of the spectrum, some EMS systems, due to financial handicaps, bureaucratic red tape, or a pervasive reluctance to abandon traditional methods and try something new, continue to conduct their dispatching functions manually.

There is absolutely nothing inherently wrong with manual dispatch systems, although it's naturally easier and faster if you can make a computer do part of the work for you; however, if you use a manual system, you should be aware of one unconditional necessity. *Status changes or the occurrence of an unusual event, request for additional resources, and the like, must be time stamped by some method that is commonly accepted as credible.* Procedures and standards for credible and reliable documentation vary in different areas of the country.

Many manual dispatch systems incorporate the use of a simple *locking* time clock; this is an easily implemented system improvement, since most providers already use this apparatus for payroll purposes. Dispatch cards are formatted to allow each card to be inserted into a mechanical time clock and stamped or punched each time a status change occurs. The information recorded on time-stamped dispatch cards will probably be viewed from a legal perspective as being more credible and reliable than handwritten information, since it is more difficult to alter a mechanically recorded time.

This recommendation applies not only to those who work with manual dispatch systems, but also to those communicators who enjoy the benefits of computer assisted dispatch. *When your CAD system is inoperable for any reason, the practice of writing in the times on a dispatch card is really not sufficient; status changes should be recorded by punching a time clock.* Obviously, this method of time-keeping is reliable only if line communicators or dispatchers cannot alter the settings of the time clock. The key should always remain secured with a communications supervisor; if adjustments to the month, day, date, or time displayed by the clock require adjustment, those corrections should be made by the supervisor, and only when the time clock is not in use to record the progression of events during an active call.

## TYPES OF REPORTING AND DOCUMENTATION: DIFFERENT NEEDS, DIFFERENT METHODS

The reporting needs of medical services generally fall into four broad subject categories: medical data, legal safeguards, maintenance of the health of the community, and information for planning, billing, and administrative purposes. In any emergency medical response system, we must provide the required information in an easily understandable and readily retrievable format. Stored information may consist of written patient encounter forms, manual run cards, written dispatch logs, consistently marked and filed audio recordings, microfilm, computer assisted dispatch systems, or free-standing personal computers and computer networks.

## Medical Information: Documentation of the Response

Most medical reporting about a particular patient is completed by the field personnel who provide the hands-on patient care. This information is written on what, in various systems, is called a patient encounter form, a run sheet, or a "street" form. However, the documentation of each response must also be executed in the communications center, *even if some effort is duplicated*. The existence of duplicate information allows additional opportunities to double-check, verify, and validate that information. A printed form, dispatch card, or computer entry screen must be organized to allow the recording of each pertinent piece of information in logical order. The elements of medical information that must be recorded in the documentation of each response, whether accomplished by field personnel, communications personnel, or both, include:

- Incident location (address)
- Response priority
- Type of incident (presumptive patient condition)
- Age, sex, and weight of patient
- Chief complaint
- Nature of illness or injury
- History of illness or mechanism of injury
- Signs and symptoms at time of initial contact, on scene, during transport, and on arrival at transport destination
- Vital signs and results of physical exam
- Care or intervention given by bystanders prior to arrival of crew
- Care given by crew
- Medications taken prior to or during event and/or administered by crew
- Changes in patient condition
- Name of patient, if applicable
- Name of person calling, if applicable
- Notifying agency
- Special scene conditions or patient requirements
- Referencing number (incident number, call number, etc.) for information retrieval purposes
- Transport destination and priority

Medical information kept on file should routinely include audio recordings demonstrating positive intervention techniques and pre-arrival instructions. Although they do not involve "hands-on" patient care, the information contained in these recordings is medical in nature. They may be used for training and retraining of the medical communicator, and for orientation and reorientation of field personnel to communications center procedures.

**Chart Audit/Incident Investigation Requests** Any medical response system or agency that strives to provide the highest quality patient care must have in place a comprehensive, carefully organized quality assurance and quality improvement program. The quality control procedures outlined in this text are structured specifically to ensure adherence to high performance standards in the communications center; they are designed to function as part of a larger, systemwide plan.

In a high-performance system, the care administered during each ambulance response should be individually reviewed. While this may, upon initial consideration, seem a monumental task, it can be accomplished through aggressive planning and thoughtful organization. Field training officers are selected through a standardized process of testing and interviews; once the selections have been made, additional training is provided to these individuals. The number of designated training officers will be dependent on the size of the system and the volume of calls run. Completed patient encounter forms are assigned in equal numbers to the trainers for their individual review and comments. Unusual, exceptional, or problem calls are referred directly to the system's clinical coordinator.

Even with a quality improvement program such as this in place, incidents will regularly occur that require more investigation than will be accomplished through routine reviewing procedures. In systems in which supervisors, managers, and administrators accept total responsibility for the actions and competency levels of their employees, chart reviews and incident investigations will be welcomed *from any source*. Procedures must be established to handle these requests for further information. Complaints or requests for further documentation and investigation of the events taking place during or surrounding a response (see Figure 14.1) may originate with anyone: concerned family members, receiving physicians, medical communicators, field personnel, hospital staff members, field supervisors, and even uninvolved bystanders. Each complaint or request must be viewed seriously and handled with courtesy and tact; each must be investigated with a completely open mind. Even if the problem is only a perceptual one, it is still a problem. *You cannot resolve a problem if you don't know it exists.*

The request to pull and review additional information about a particular call should always be conscientiously accepted, and the documentation package (written reports or audio tapes) completed in a timely manner. However, the security and confidentiality of these records is defined in many different ways, and the determination is influenced by current national, state, and local trends and standards. Therefore, the release of information must be carefully controlled. For example, in some service areas, audio tapes are considered to be part of the public record, and therefore may be accessed by anyone. Conversely, hard-copy documentation (including both manual dispatch cards and CAD-generated run reports) is frequently judged to be part of the confidential patient record, and a subpoena is required before the record can be released.

| | | |
|---|---|---|
| SERVICE INQUIRY/COMPLAINT<br>REQUEST FOR CHART AUDIT/INCIDENT INVESTIGATION |||
| Date of Service 2/10 | Date of Inquiry 2/16 | Invoice Number 1902 |
| Encounter Address 3132 North Main |||
| Patient Name James Anderson || Telephone Number 555-6163 |
| Name of Person Initiating Inquiry/Complaint Helen Anderson |||
| Relationship to Patient Wife |||
| Has Patient Signed Authorization to Release Information? Yes |||
| Nature and Specifics of Inquiry/Complaint<br>Wife says she specifically requested a non-Emergency response, yet an Emergency ambulance was sent — |||
| Approximate Time of Incident 0635 |||
| Information/Data Requested<br>☑ Printed Copy: CAD Generated Run Report<br>☑ Printed Copy: Patient Encounter Form<br>☑ Printed Copy: Transaction Logging Record<br>☑ Audio Tape: Incoming request for service/triage |||
| Incident Investigated by S. Smith || Department Comms. |
| Findings: Caller did request non-Emergency ambulance. She then stated her husband was having chest pain and some shortness of breath. Call was correctly prioritized + correctly dispatched. |||
| Findings Reported To David Johnson MD/Med. Dir || Date 2/18 |
| Report Made By S. Smith |||

Figure 14.1 *Service inquiry*

Because of these variables, a standardized procedure must be established which allows for the *controlled* release of information. The information package that results from a chart audit or investigation request should be routinely routed to one person or position within the organization who will review the incident and make the information available to the person or agency requesting the audit.

Legal Documentation

A wide range of recorded information is necessary to fulfill the requirements for adequate legal documentation. This data can be used to substantiate billing procedures, show a sequence of events, or justify a series of actions. The ability to retrieve this information will allow you to explain or justify the actions taken by members of your department in questionable situations, and to defend yourself and other medical communicators against charges of unsound practices. This data will also enable you to provide an accurate and complete narrative if you are called to testify during criminal proceedings. Audio recordings of telephone calls for help often contain information about the circumstances leading up to and during the commission of violent crimes, confessions, and dying statements. As the medical communicator becomes more visible to the public and more widely recognized as an active participant in the administration of patient care, medical dispatchers will be called upon more frequently to provide historical information in cases of both criminal and civil litigation.

**Response Information** Elements that must be included to provide an accurate and complete written or printed legal record of any response include:

- Date of request for service
- Date of response
- Name/ID of call-taker
- City, response area, or district in which incident address is located
- Type of incident (patient condition category)
- Special patient requirements
- Time unit dispatched
- ID of all responding units
- ID of personnel on responding units
- Time first responders were requested
- Time first responders arrived on scene
- Time original ambulance arrived on scene
- Time patient transport began
- Destination/priority changes

- Time of request for service
- Scheduled pick-up time
- Incident location address
- Call-back numbers
- Caller's name
- Patient's name
- Notifying agency
- Special scene conditions
- Referencing (run) number
- Name/ID of dispatcher
- Time unit responded
- Location from which unit responded
- Time law enforcement was requested
- Time law enforcement arrived on scene
- Time medical information relayed to hospital
- Transport destination
- Transport priority

- Reasons for destination or priority changes
- Time of arrival at destination
- Reason for extended drop time at destination
- Explanation of any unusual occurrence during call
- Time unit canceled
- Name of person or agency canceling response
- Total response time (time call received to time first ambulance on scene)
- All applicable times for all additional responding ambulances
- Reasons for response or transport changes
- Time unit available for emergency response
- Time unit became mobile from destination
- Time patient refused treatment/transportation
- Reason for cancellation
- Reason for patient non-transport
- Compliance or non-compliance with contracted response time requirements
- Factors contributing to non-compliant response time

Whether response documentation is accomplished manually or through the use of a CAD system, the data in each field of each completed dispatch card or report must be visually verified. This task is usually performed by the communicator who dispatched the response. Each communicator should "sign off" on each response, signifying that she/he has verified the validity of the information, and that she/he accepts responsibility for its accuracy.

**Optimal Structure and Use of Audio Recording Systems**
Although many types of recording systems are used in medical communications centers, the most efficient setups include the following components:

- Voice-activated cassette recording units mounted in each radio and telephone console, capable of instantaneous playback
- A "master" recorder capable of 24-hour continuous recording of all radio and telephone traffic with back-up and fail-safe features
- If the master recorder utilizes reel-to-reel tapes, enough tapes are necessary to allow audio records to be kept for a realistic period of time before the tapes are recycled and recorded over
- A playback unit with digital time readout which operates separately from and/or concurrently with the master recorder

Many public safety communications centers utilize multiple-cassette recording and playback systems. While these are generally much less expensive than the larger reel-to-reel units, there are potential problems inherent with multiple-cassette systems of which the communicator should be aware. First, the quality of sound is sometimes less than optimal on recordings made from cassette units. Second, even large multiple-cassette recorders may require more on-shift maintenance than reel-to-reel units. The tapes on intelligently selected reel-to-reel systems need only be changed once in a 24-hour period, while some cassette units require tape changes as often as once per hour. And third, reel-to-reel tapes which play back sound in "real time" would logically be considered credible, and as such, are admissible in court; although procedures vary by state and type of litigation, cassette tapes, because of the ease with which they can be altered, are sometimes considered less reliable and may not be credible as evidence. One advantage of using a cassette system is the immediate accessibility of the recordings.

In cases where information received by the medical dispatcher will be used as evidence in a criminal proceeding (child abuse, homicide, suicide, etc.), specific security measures are indicated. Again, procedures and precedents are determined by local and state standards. One method of securing the recordings is to place the reel-to-reel master tape in the possession of a specific law enforcement official, or a person in a position within the EMS system specifically designated to fulfill that function. The person charged with this task must receive special instruction from law enforcement personnel in methods of securing evidence and establishing a chain of evidence.

Charges that a medical dispatcher took inappropriate action can come from many different sources, and accusations may vary from simple billing disputes to nonemergency service delays to allegations that the communicator's behavior actually caused or contributed to the death or serious injury of a patient. *Every complaint, whether critical or noncritical, must be individually and completely addressed. Every negative impression left with a client must be corrected to a positive one.*

At one time, it was believed that the existence of audio recordings could actually be detrimental to the defense of the medical communicator against complaining parties. If no tape existed, then the problem would eventually come down to "Our word against theirs." Again, times have changed, and standards have changed with them. It is now routine procedure not only to consistently conform to high performance standards, but to provide proof that you have done so. If a system's dispatch personnel are comprehensively trained and their performance regularly reviewed, that system has nothing to fear and everything to gain by providing audible evidence in any dispute.

Voice-activated recording and playback devices mounted at each console position enable both call-taker and radio operator to instantly play back any questionable voice transmission. If, for example, a field unit voices a message that is unreadable to the radio operator, she/he can rewind the tape and quickly listen again to the transmission, reviewing it for content. If a unit arriving in an apartment complex on an emergency response voices difficulty in locating the patient, the call-taker can immediately review her/his tape to confirm the building designation and apartment number.

**Recording System Operation** With all the elements of the above-outlined system in place, all telephone lines and radio channels in use in the system should be connected to designated recording channels within the master recorder, which runs constantly, 24 hours a day. In each 24-hour period, ideally during times of predictably low call volume, completed tapes are rewound, removed, and stored, and blank tapes are inserted into the recorder. Recorded tapes are numbered and filed for reference until the entire stock of blank tapes has been exhausted. At that time, previously recorded tapes are recorded over in numerical order, unless a particular tape has been secured as evidence in a criminal proceeding by order of a law enforcement agency.

**Time Constraints for Civil Litigation** Working as a medical communicator, you are constantly exposed to the risk of civil litigation. Risk factors and legal principles as they apply to medical services are detailed in Chapter 13. However, the time constraints that apply to civil actions *must* be considered when initiating, restructuring, or evaluating any system of recordkeeping and documentation.

Most states have established limited time periods within which those persons filing civil actions must operate. These time limits differ from state to state. In some states, a civil action must be filed within a time period not to exceed 2 years from the date of the causative event; in others, the time limit is one year, or one year and one day. Many, many times, a civil action will be filed only days or hours before the end of the established time period. *Don't kid yourself: This is not an accident.* It is a litigation technique that has been tested and has repeatedly been proven effective. As the attorneys delay filing the action, their chances of winning their case increase. If an action is not filed until 2 years after a particular incident took place, an additional 3 years *or more* may elapse before the case actually comes to trial. Considering the filing delay, the length of time required for routine notification and subpoena processes, jury selection, and court docket delays and postponements, it is easily conceivable that the elapsed time between when you received or dispatched a call and when you are required to appear in court to defend yourself against civil claims related to that call can be *5 to 10 years*. In a highly productive system, you may receive and dispatch literally hundreds of thousands of calls in that length of time. The longer the actual trial date can be postponed, the better the chance is that you will not remember the incident, or will not be able to produce definitive documentation to defend yourself. *Every plan for recordkeeping, documentation, and the filing and retrieval of information must be structured with the possibility of defense against civil litigation in mind.*

**No Transports and Unit Cancellations** Any time an ambulance response is initiated and no patient is transported, careful documentation must be completed. Remember that the most common scenario in which charges are brought against an ambulance provider is the situation where either no ambulance was sent, or no patient was transported. In different systems, these incidents are called, for example, dry runs, no-rides, canceled runs. Various circumstances may surround this type of event: the ambulance may be canceled by any number of persons or agencies while still responding to the call; the first responder agency or company may arrive on the scene and recognize that there is no need for the ambulance to continue its response; the ambulance crew may arrive to find that the patient has already left the scene; the request for an ambulance response may have been made by a concerned third party when no real need existed; the ambulance may arrive on scene to find a patient who refuses treatment or transportation; and so on.

It is critically important that each system standardize its own list of reasons for dry runs. In most systems, these reasons are coded, either to allow an active call to be canceled through a CAD system, or to decrease the space used to note the cancellation reason on a manual dispatch card. *Any time a response is begun and no patient transport results, the reason for the dry run or cancellation must be carefully and accurately noted.*

Some of the most common reasons for nontransport of a patient are:

- Closer unit sent
- Higher priority call
- Calling party canceled
- Unit on scene canceled
- Police canceled
- Fire canceled
- Police transported
- Fire transported
- Vehicle mechanical failure
- Patient left scene before arrival of ambulance
- Duplicate call
- Unable to locate (false call)
- Dead on scene
- Patient refused
- No sick or injured
- Other unit transported
- Other service transported
- Helicopter transported
- Other equipment failure

The reason for each patient nontransport must be *very precisely* noted on the communications form or dispatch card. For example, "Unable to locate" and "Patient left scene before arrival of ambulance" will be interpreted differently in a court of law, and "No sick or injured" is distinctly different from "Patient refused treatment or transport" as an incident disposition. *Each reason given in the permanent record for the nontransport of a patient should correspond with the reason given by the voice signal on the audio tape, whether the voice signal was made by the radio operator canceling a unit en route or a field crew member clearing the scene of an incident.*

**Patient Refusals** As with unit cancellations, patient refusals must be handled with special care. A common practice is to stock standardized patient refusal release forms (reviewed and approved by the system's legal counsel) as part of the routine paperwork package carried by each crew and/or on each ambulance. To provide an additional level of documentation and an additional measure of protection, a further procedure should be established.

When *any* patient contact is made and the patient refuses treatment and/or transport by ambulance, the particulars of the patient's condition and the circumstances surrounding the refusal should be documented *in detail*. This should be accomplished both on the written patient encounter form and by a voice recording on an audio tape. The designated primary care-giver on the unit involved should use whatever mechanism (*recorded* telephone lines or radio channels) is normally used to transmit direct-voice patient reports to base station hospitals. If the field care-giver is not uncomfortable with the patient refusal, she/he may simply request to document the refusal with communications center personnel. She/he should give a complete and accurate accounting of conditions found, the chief complaint, the patient's condition, signs and symptoms, pertinent medical history or mechanism of injury, vital signs, results of the physical exam, any unusual factors, the patient's reasons for refusing treatment and/or transport, whether or not the patient has read and signed the AMA (against medical advice) form, and whether or not the patient has been advised of the possible negative consequences of not seeking medical attention. When the report is complete, an advisory statement should be repeated to the care-giver. An example of typical phrasing is, "If the patient is conscious, alert, and oriented, understands the seriousness of his condition, and has read and signed the AMA form, then he has the legal right to refuse. Please advise the patient again that we still recommend he see a physician. The time of refusal is 1645." Another option is to read a similar statement to the patient herself/himself, and have the patient's voice recorded on tape refusing transport.

In *any* case where the communicator is not comfortable with the refusal circumstances or situation (when there has been a loss of consciousness, when the patient's condition is obviously unstable, etc.), the field care-giver should be connected with or patched through to a base physician, using whatever mechanism is in place to provide direct voice contact between field crews and base hospitals.

While any patient who is conscious, alert, and oriented to person, place, time, and event has the legal right to refuse service, the EMS provider also has the right to secure whatever legal protection can be made available.

**Unusual Incident Reporting** Any time an unusual event occurs, an uncommon set of circumstances surrounds a response, or a complaint is made about the behavior of a medical dispatcher or field care-giver, the communicators involved in or witnessing the event must complete documentation of the occurrence. Unusual incidents may involve communicator errors (dispatch delays, wrong unit sent, etc.), problems among responding agencies (jurisdictional disputes, poor resource allocation), and complaints from family members (charges of lack of telephone courtesy, questions about patient care or response times).

A standardized Unusual Incident Reporting form (see Figure 14.2) should be made available to help the communicator document information about the event. All pertinent dates, times, and other information required in the documentation of any response must be included. When possible, a photocopy of the hard-copy documentation (CAD-generated run sheet or manual dispatch card) should be attached.

Part of any manager's or supervisor's job is to research allegations of inappropriate actions, and to document responses to those

Chap. 14    Documentation and Reporting Techniques    **141**

| UNUSUAL INCIDENT REPORT ||
|---|---|
| Report To S. Smith | Department Comms |
| Report From B. Adams | Department Operations |
| Date Rec'd 2/11    By S. Smith | Reply Requested? No/FYI |
| Date of Incident 2/10 | Time of Incident 0635 |
| Communicators Involved ? ||
| Field Crew Members Involved/Unit Numbers Medic 20 - Baker + Green ||
| Other Personnel/Agencies Involved B. Adams/Field Operation Supervisor ||
| Invoice/Incident Number(s) 1902 ||
| Description of Events On this date, Medic 20 requested that I meet them at All Saints Hospital. Family members of their patient were very upset, as they had requested a transfer ambulance + Medic 20 arrived with lights + siren.<br><br>B. Adams ||

Figure 14.2  *Unusual incident report*

charges. To accomplish these tasks, the communications administrator must have a timely awareness of unusual events. This is most easily accomplished when unusual incident reports are filled out by the communicators on duty before they terminate their shifts. Remember, your memory is unreliable; it may distort your perceptions of any incident if you wait days, or even hours, before you write it up.

Maintaining Community Health

Medical communicators can contribute to the overall health and safety of the citizens in their service areas by keeping accurate records and establishing efficient notification practices when certain types of events or situations occur. Information files can be amassed detailing known scene hazards of specific addresses (chemicals routinely stored in businesses, radiation risks, fire hazards, etc.). Local health departments can be warned of suspected instances of food poisoning. Animal control officers can be apprised of responses involving animal bites. All these pieces of information can improve the well-being of the community and aid the medical response system in providing the highest quality patient care, while helping to ensure the safety of responding units.

**Between a Rock and a Hard Place** Aggressive new educational programs and system performance requirements are emerging daily as part of the national effort to limit exposure to communicable diseases. At one time, the existence of policies and procedures to safeguard employee health and well-being was exceptional, and was seen as the mark of a caring employer. These procedures are now the law.

In trying to responsibly address this problem, the medical communicator finds herself/himself occupying a difficult position. Should you protect patient confidentiality and risk exposing your field personnel to catastrophic illness? Should you transmit information that will limit your field crews' risk of exposure, but will destroy the privacy of the patient? Which choice is legally the safest? *Which is right?*

The risk of exposure to communicable diseases such as meningitis and hepatitis has always been a cause for concern. With the added threat of the HIV virus, making the correct choice becomes ultimately critical, since mistakes can literally be fatal.

On one hand, the HIV+ patient has the same rights to privacy as the patient with hepatitis. If patient confidentiality is violated, the danger for the HIV+ patient is even greater than for patients with other communicable diseases; if the knowledge of this patient's illness is made public, she/he may be fired from a job, have the lease to an apartment canceled without warning, or find that she/he suddenly has no medical insurance. *These are real people we're talking about here.* The HIV+ patient has already been diagnosed as having an illness that is degenerative, painful, incredibly expensive, and invariably fatal. If we can possibly avoid adding to this patient's problems, we must do so. Aside from the very real hardships caused to this patient when confidentiality is breached, the communicator and the system may be sued to compensate the patient for losses resulting from the dispatcher's actions.

Our counterparts who provide field care believe, without exception, that they are entitled to know when the threat of exposure to a catastrophic disease is a possibility. While, as medical professionals, we are all aware of various rules and regulations established to limit our risks when providing direct-contact patient care (putting on gloves before contacting body fluids, maintaining aseptic technique), *what if the care-giver forgets*? Receiving a supervisory reprimand may not be the only consequence of making this type of error; the field crew member may actually develop a serious or fatal illness. As medical dispatchers and system status controllers, we are morally, ethically, and professionally accountable for the safety of our field personnel. If we do not warn our personnel of a possible risk, aren't we at least partially culpable if our personnel do contract the disease?

The truly responsible resolution of this dilemma lies in a compromise between the two choices clearly defined earlier. Patients are entitled to privacy; care-givers are entitled to protect themselves. What solution will answer to the needs of both?

Premise history or hazardous locations files should be accumulated, updated, and maintained in a timely manner. These files may consist of paper forms stored in alphabetical order in a filing cabinet, information cards arranged by district in a card file, or collections of data electronically recorded in a computer program within the CAD system. Any method that allows for easy access and rapid retrieval of the data is acceptable. *The most critical factor is the manner in which the information is documented.*

**Communicable Diseases** Here are some basic guidelines to help you in documenting possible risks for exposure to communicable diseases:

> You *should* "flag" the address as having a premise history or known scene hazard.
>
> You *should* document that any responders to the address must take sterile precautions or universal precautions.
>
> You *should* advise the responding crews over a radio channel to *"Take sterile precautions"* or *"Take universal precautions."*
>
> You *should not* identify the specific disease from which the patient suffers in your premise history file.
>
> You *should not* broadcast statements such as, "This is a known AIDS patient," or "This patient has infectious hepatitis."

When a specific policy has been drafted, reviewed by legal counsel, and implemented, there will no longer be a need to broadcast specific information over radio channels accessible to the public. Your field crews will understand exactly what is meant by the general warning, and will be reminded to protect themselves.

### Physical Scene Hazards and Litigation Considerations

Chemical, radiation, and fire hazards are usually straightforward and easily documented. If, for example, a particular chemical is stored on the premises in question, you can safely keep records saying so; and, as long as the information is strictly factual, you can transmit the nature of the hazards over the radio. However, premise histories that refer to persons rather than things must be handled with extreme caution.

Here's an example: Last year, you sent a unit to a reported medical emergency at a residential address. When the crew arrived on the scene, they encountered a hostile and violent man who repeatedly screamed unintelligible words and phrases at them. He then attacked the crew with a baseball bat, injuring the paramedic. You requested a police department response. When the police arrived, they handcuffed the man and placed him in custody. You had to dispatch a field supervisor and two other EMS units, one to transport the man to the hospital for psychiatric evaluation, and one to transport the paramedic. Your crew members later told you the man was nuts; the police department dispatcher told you her officers thought he was under the influence of PCP or some other drug.

Obviously, this address should somehow be flagged; no communicator should unknowingly send another EMS crew to this location without simultaneously dispatching the police department and advising all responding units of the possible dangers. However, the *content* of the information must be carefully worded. This is an example of an inappropriate premise history:

> "Psychotic male resident, hostile to police and EMS crews. Patient is extremely violent. Narcotics involved."

The recording or transmission of this type of grossly subjective information is a very unsound practice. Nothing that took place during the previous incident factually or medically establishes that this patient is "psychotic"; "hostile" and "extremely violent" are subjective terms that are not easy to clearly define; and the only person who suggested that drugs were involved never directly interacted with the patient. This type of information can be held to be slanderous, and as such, may be actionable. When a later response is made to this address, the allegation may also be made that this information prejudiced communicators and care-givers before the unit arrived on the scene, and that this prejudice delayed the response or had a negative impact on the care given. Risky, risky practice.

Here is an example of appropriate documentation of the above situation:

> "35–45 year old male in residence 12/30/89 struck EMS personnel with wooden baseball bat. Dispatch PD. Instruct crew not to enter the residence without police officers."

This is factual information which identifies an actual occurrence; the events can be substantiated by the police report filed after the original incident. Precise instructions are provided for responding personnel. No statements or insinuations are made about the character of the resident. No name is given, and no racial information is provided. No reference at all is made about the resident's mental status, or the possibility of drug usage. The date of the previous incident is noted; this is important information. If considerable time has passed since the identification date of a specific scene hazard, the hazard may not still exist at the time of any subsequent dispatch. A resident who previously caused a problem may no longer live at the address. A business that stored volatile chemicals may have relocated to another part of the service area. Information may be associated with the current occupant (who is now your patient), when the precautionary statements actually referred to a person who moved away from the address months or years ago, or who is now deceased.

When a crew responds to an address with a specific premise history, request that they provide you with follow-up information. Using the updated data, you can periodically review your files and purge them of obsolete information.

### Recording Data for Administrative Purposes

Administrative documentation needs vary with the variety of the system in place and the structure and organization of that system. Some reports that are consistently used even in different types of provider systems are:

- Run reports: used to establish a series of events; to prove that service was provided, thereby justifying patient billing; to provide basic information from which to build a complete accounting of any incident; etc.
- Scheduling and staffing records: used for payroll
- Response time reports: to demonstrate to customers, clients, and governing agencies the provider's compliance with contract requirements
- Elapsed call time reports: to show the average length of time required to complete calls of all priorities; to ensure that total average call time does not exceed one hour
- Drop time reports: to demonstrate the average length of time spent by field crews at receiving facilities; to identify the causes of extended drop times (whether individual field employees, times of day, or inefficient procedures at specific receiving facilities), and to correct problems and potential problems
- Unit hour utilization reports: used to prove the percentage of time that each shift type is actually productive; to project future incomes; to maintain a financial balance
- Call volume reports: used in system status management to predict future call demands, and to plan for staffing; to predict exact dates when new employees will need to be trained and ready to work; to time training schools and academies to be complete

*before* a staffing "crunch" occurs; to show annual or seasonal call volume increases; to justify budget needs; to increase the size of the fleet; etc.

- Lost/added unit hour reports: to document available unit hours taken from or added to scheduled unit hours during a particular time period; to identify the causes of unit hour losses (downtime for emergency vehicle maintenance, personnel tardiness or absences, etc.) or added unit hours (to identify instances of poor planning), and to reduce future instances of deviation from the planned schedule
- Equipment downtime reports: to identify obsolete or worn out equipment (including everything from ambulances to radio equipment to computers) so repair procedures may be improved or the equipment replaced

These are just a few of the reports generated by medical service providers nationwide. The actual reports vary between service areas and types of systems (fire department EMS, private sector EMS, cross-trained public safety departments, third city services, etc.). Samples of specific reporting forms are provided in this manuscript under related chapter headings.

## THE COMMITMENT TO EXCELLENCE

Records can be maintained in many forms, and the information utilized in many ways, but one requirement remains constant: *The information must consistently be absolutely, totally, completely, indisputably accurate.*

*If your service is to be successful, if you are to enjoy professional respect, a good reputation, and financial prosperity, your service will have to compete in a free marketplace against many other systems.* You, as a medical communicator, may not be employed by a privately owned EMS company. You may work for a fire service, or for a city government; if so, it may be that your system will never be required to compete for a specific *contract*. However, whether you like it or not, you do have to compete for media attention, positive feedback, budget funds, and professional respect. The only way to successfully compete in the EMS marketplace is to set high performance standards (for both patient care and financial efficiency), *and then prove that you can live up to them*. That proof is provided concretely both to your public and to your fellow professionals in the form of reports, published studies, and confirmed improvements resulting from procedural changes. *All of these are types of documentation.*

"Garbage in, garbage out." Say that several times to yourself. The results of your analyses, your planning, and your diagrams for future improvements and innovations will be only as valid as the original reports from which your information base is built. If the original data is incorrect, the end product will be invalid, and without value. Make the commitment now to refine and streamline your reporting procedures, and to provide the most complete and accurate documentation possible.

## SUMMARY AND REVIEW

1. Why is accurate documentation and recordkeeping even more important now than in years past?

2. How can audio recordings be used as documentation?

3. Which type of recording mechanism is preferable? Why?

4. What are the advantages of a multiple-cassette recording system?

5. What are the four basic types of documentation needed in the field of emergency pre-hospital care?

6. List 15 information items typically included in the documentation of any response.

7. What purpose do chart audit and incident investigation requests serve?

8. What types of information will provide you with some measure of legal protection?

9. What kind of recording system does your communications center have in place? How could the system be improved?

10. What are the time constraints in your area for civil litigation?

11. What type of documentation should be completed when "No transports," unit cancellations, and patient refusals occur?

12. How can good recordkeeping contribute to maintaining community health?

# Chapter 15

# PUBLIC RELATIONS

*"Public opinion is stronger than the legislature,
and nearly as strong as the ten commandments."*
— *Charles Dudley Warner,* My Summer in a Garden

*"A word is dead when it is said, some say.
I say it just begins to live that day."*
— *Emily Dickinson,* Part I, Life

## WHAT IS IT? (WHAT ARE THEY?): A QUESTION OF SEMANTICS

Public relations is the planned effort to influence public opinion, action, and reaction through examples of good character and demonstration of responsible performance. Public relations is dynamic; it moves. It adapts itself to change as the demands placed upon it change.

Public relations consists of those functions concerned with informing the public of an organization's activities, capabilities, and policies, and attempting to create a favorable public opinion of these. The need for a solid, capable public relations campaign in any emergency medical service, whether city-funded or privately owned, is obvious; so are the complex demands that will be placed on such a program.

A workable, effective public relations program for an EMS system incorporates all the characteristics just mentioned; it also plans its actions in ways that promote good will, empathy, understanding, respect, and even compromise, when indicated. The various components of an EMS public relations plan include everything from costly mass media events to the most basic policies and procedures of the service.

There are three common ways in which medical dispatchers can impact the public's image of EMS workers: by the manner in which they deal with the media, by creating and participating in public education programs, and by the nature of their efforts in the area of total customer satisfaction.

## DEALING WITH THE MEDIA: THE NATURE OF THE PROCESS

*"There's no point in making noises if no one is listening."*
— *Duke Ellington*

The total effectiveness of any public relations approach is based on communication. Each day, the medical communicator acts as a critical player in the information exchange that enables the field care-giver to provide high-quality patient care and customer satisfaction. Although acting as an effective medical communicator is difficult, the fact that we can accomplish the function *at all* is due to the common knowledge and language we share with our co-workers in the field.

When we attempt to relay understandable information to those outside our industry, the process becomes much more complicated.

One of the ways in which the medical dispatcher participates in the public relations effort is in dealing with the media. When a media representative calls to request information about a current or past call or event, the dispatcher relays selected information to her/him. Many people involved in the relay of information mistakenly believe that their responsibility lies only in selecting and stating the information to be relayed. However, this only works if the persons sending and receiving the information have a common knowledge base or frame of reference.

### Back to Basic Communication

The three fundamental elements in the relay of information are the sender, the message, and the receiver. These components interact with other elements in what is basically a repeating circular pattern (see Figure 15.1).

### Changing Your Attitude Toward Media Representatives

When you are working in the communications center, you are dealing with life and death on a daily basis. You know how important your job is; you are also constantly aware of how time-critical your actions are. You continuously reprioritize all the information around you; vitally important matters are dealt with immediately and with a high degree of attention. Insignificant items are put on hold, or invested with a minimum of personal attention. At some point, unless you prepare for the phenomenon and take steps to avoid it, you will begin to apply this prioritization process to every action you perform and every piece of sensory information you receive, *critical or noncritical, work-related or not.*

```
┌─────────────────┐
│ The event or source │
│ of information is   │
│ decoded by the      │
│ sender into an      │
│ understandable form │
└─────────────────┘
```

```
┌──────────────┐         ┌──────────────┐
│ Understandable│         │ Understandable│
│ information   │         │ information   │
│ is used       │         │ is encoded by │
│ or relayed    │         │ the sender into│
│ again         │         │ the message   │
└──────────────┘         └──────────────┘
```

```
┌──────────────┐         ┌──────────────┐
│ The receiver │         │ The          │
│ decodes the  │         │ sender       │
│ message into an│       │ sends        │
│ understandable│        │ the          │
│ form         │         │ message      │
└──────────────┘         └──────────────┘
```

```
┌──────────────┐
│ The          │
│ message      │
│ is received  │
│ by the       │
│ receiver     │
└──────────────┘
```

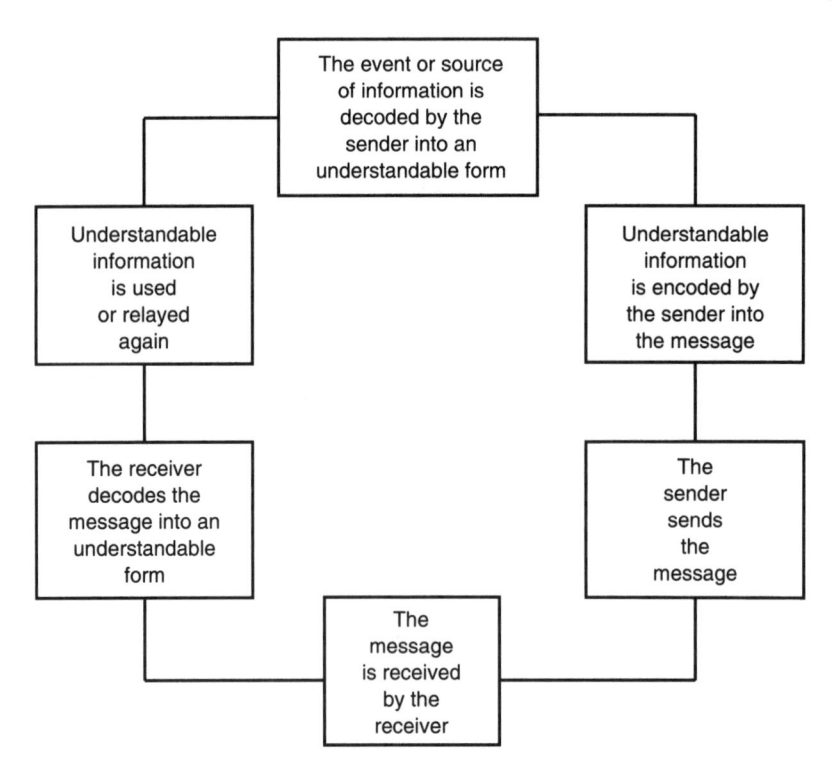

Figure 15.1  *Basic communication*

Employees in emergency medical service have traditionally regarded representatives of the media with an almost schizophrenic perspective. From one angle, we have viewed media personnel with comparatively low esteem. Reporters seldom do things the way we want them done; they report incidents differently than the way we remember them. They misspell our names and identify us as fire department personnel when we are employees of a private service, and as "ambulance drivers" when we work for a fire department. Since we, as a group, tend to be inordinately proud of the services we provide, these errors contribute to our lack of respect for media reps in general.

On the other hand, when we participate in a heroic life-saving attempt, we want their attention, and we want it now. We are flattered by the media exposure; since very few people actually understand and appreciate the job we do, it feels good to occasionally receive broad-based recognition for our efforts. When we participate in what we consider to be a "newsworthy" event, we virtually demand that the incident be given fast, extensive coverage and exposure.

When the typical medical dispatcher receives a telephone request from a media representative for information about a call, she/he usually views the entire conversation as an irritant. We are busy. It's none of their business. We have more important things to do than talk to a reporter on the telephone. We also, as a group, become possessive and protective of "our" crews, "our" patients, and "our" system. While these feelings are a natural derivation from the intense sense of responsibility connected with the communicator's job, they are frequently displayed in a manner that is inappropriate.

As has been suggested before in this document, you're smart people. *Figure it out.* These are not machines we are dealing with; they are people who happen to have chosen for their life's work the publication of news, just as we chose EMS. When we deal with people, we also deal with their attitudes and egos. We cannot display terse, abrupt, uncooperative, or rude telephone behavior to media people one day, and expect them to welcome the opportunity to provide us with positive, free, image-enhancing publicity the next. *The exchange of information with the media has to be a two-way street. These callers are also entitled to the same respect and courtesy you show to any citizen in your service area who places a nonemergency call to gather any type of information.*

Practical Guidelines for Release of Information

Even when you have adjusted your own mind-set and want to build a cooperative relationship with your local media personnel, these questions still arise: *What information can you appropriately release for possible publication or broadcast? What information should be kept confidential?*

Check with your management or command staff; also solicit the opinion and advice of your system's legal counsel. In most areas, this is an acceptable basic rule for what data you can provide to anyone who calls requesting it:

> You can release to any media representative any item of information that was broadcast over your dispatch channels.

Since anything broadcast over your dispatch channels is, in a sense, already public information, you will usually not place yourself at risk if you relay the information further. The information is already accessible to any citizen who has a scanner and a list of the frequencies in use in your area. *Any item of information that falls outside this clear delineation may, at a later time, be categorized as confidential patient information, and probably should not be passed on.*

Major Media Events

When an incident occurs that requires an unusually large or complicated response, involves unusual circumstances, and so on, you may receive a number of media calls in the dispatch center. While these calls are of lower priority than calls affecting patient care, crew safety, or customer service, it is still in the best interest of your system that they be handled efficiently and politely.

In an unusual incident as described previously, the communicator should offer the acting media liaison for the system the opportunity to contact the media directly, thus providing her/him with the opening to direct and/or limit the flow of information, make position statements, and the like. Your system's public relations officer or public information officer will usually have her or his own established contacts within the media work force. She or he should know, for example, which reporters can be relied on to report accurately, which are sympathetic and unsympathetic to your system's position, etc. Therefore, the most efficient way in which to provide other agencies with information is usually to have your public relations officer contact media representatives directly. Notify your PR officer of the unusual incident, providing her or him with the location, times, and pertinent details of the event. *Make sure your information is correct.* (This system of relaying information won't survive long if you make your own personnel look like fools.) Then allow the system representative to decide which media people to contact, and what to tell them.

When major or unusual incidents occur, it may be in your best interest to have your public information officer come to the communications center and field media calls directly.

## PUBLIC EDUCATION

Those of us who work in EMS routinely see people in the worst of circumstances. When it's your business to encounter unexpected situations, it becomes second nature to obsessively plan for every eventuality. Very few of us who work in this industry can delude ourselves into believing that "bad things will never happen to us." We spend a lot of time asking ourselves and each other, "What if?" We ask ourselves, "If this thing or that thing happened, what would we do? Where would we go? Who would we call?"

### The Lack of Citizen Planning

One of the things I find most fascinating about emergency medical service is the total lack of consideration given to the subject by the average citizen. Many people have no idea what kind of emergency medical help is available in their area, or how to contact and request that help. They just don't think to find out. Here are some examples of this phenomenon which I have personally encountered:

- A 45-year-old woman is diagnosed as having a degenerative heart disease, and is identified as a candidate for a heart transplant. Her family is clearly told that she may have a serious or fatal heart attack while waiting for a compatible donor organ to become available.

  Two years later, still with no donor available, the patient begins experiencing chest pain at home. She rapidly loses consciousness and falls to the floor. In the house with the patient are her husband, her adult sister, and her four children, ranging in age from 15 to 21 years. *Not one of these family members has taken instruction in CPR.*

  The husband, who calls for the ambulance, is upset and hostile; he refuses to accept CPR instruction from the call-taker. Including the time that elapsed between when the patient stopped breathing and when the husband called for help, the patient is down for 12 minutes before care-givers arrive on the scene. Although the first responders and advanced life support team have excellent response times and do everything medically indicated, the patient dies.

- A 34-year-old single mother of three children, ages 3 to 7, is diagnosed as having cancer of the brain. Her doctors prescribe an aggressive treatment program which includes radiation and chemotherapy; she continues to live at home while undergoing therapy. The ambulance crew which usually provides the patient with transportation to and from the treatment facility is impressed by the courage of both the patient and her children. The field personnel become emotionally involved in the case.

  When 3 days pass without a call for transport service from the patient, the field crew members stop by her address to check on her welfare. Through the front window of the house, the medics can see the three children huddled on the living room floor. The door is locked. After much coaxing and reassurance from the field crew, the children open the door.

  The medics find their patient slumped over the kitchen table; she is dead. The post mortem reveals that the patient choked to death; a large piece of meat has totally obstructed her airway. The cancer appears to have been in remission. The children, who are separated and placed in foster homes, did not call for help *because they didn't know how*.

- An elderly gentleman attempts to call the paramedics for his wife, who is having problems breathing. He dials the seven-digit number on the sticker he placed on his telephone more than 15 years ago. A recording tells him the number has been disconnected; although he does not know it, that ambulance service has been out of business for several years.

  The caller tries to look up "Ambulance Service" in the telephone book. His wife is gasping now and he can't find the phone number. Finally, in frustration, he dials the operator. The gentleman is so upset that he cannot tell the operator his address. She notes the caller's telephone number and calls the EMS provider for him.

  Communications center personnel check their criss-cross file to locate an address for the caller's phone number. The number is not listed.

  The emergency medical dispatcher must now place a series of calls to the security division of the local telephone company. Finally, the phone company supervisor calls back and provides the address which corresponds to the phone number given. The call is finally entered and dispatched; the medical communicator calls the elderly gentleman back to provide reassurance and pre-arrival instructions. He is now completely out of control and cannot follow the dispatcher's directions. When field care-givers arrive on the scene, the patient is in respiratory arrest. Cardiac arrest follows, and all resuscitative attempts fail. *An enhanced*

*9-1-1 system has been operational in this service area for more than a year.*

Three deaths: all tragic, and all unnecessary. In all three of these cases, the outcome could have been positive if the private citizens involved had anticipated a medical emergency. If they had taken the time to find out about their emergency medical response system, *all three patients might have survived.*

How depressing; but wait, there's more bad news. No matter how motivated you are to inform the public about the ways to access your system and the range of services you can provide, you are taking on a *very* difficult job. It's only fair that you understand what you're up against before you begin.

## Common Barriers to Change

There are many elements in human behavior that obstruct the changing process. Some are based in *understanding,* and some are issues of *control.* These are only some of the reasons why public information and educational campaigns often fail:

- *Many people only hear and retain information that agrees with and supports beliefs they already hold.* They avoid or ignore information that conflicts with their pre-existing attitudes.
- *Vocabularies and frames of reference differ.* Information intended to educate must be presented in a form your audience can understand.
- *The abilities of audience groups to understand differ.* You have to explain a thing one way to a group of first-graders, and another way to a group of businesspeople.
- *Each individual hears, interprets, and remembers an event or a message differently.* Language, cultural characteristics, peer pressure, and pre-existing educational levels can all alter a listener's perception of what is real or true.
- *Large numbers of people freely admit that they simply don't care to learn.* This is part of the process of escaping from conflict. Many people believe that they don't need this information, because the situation will never happen to them.

Aldo Leopold was one of this country's first ecologists. Early in his career as an activist, he believed that *"if the public were told how much harm ensues from unwise land use, it would mend its ways."* Later in his life, he realized that his original belief had been based on three assumptions which were simply not true:

- That the public is listening or can be made to listen;
- That the public responds, or can be made to respond, to fear of harm; and

- That ways can be mended without any important change in the public itself.[1]

Why Bother?

After digesting the previous paragraphs, you may now well believe that the general public you serve is made up of people who are ignorant, stupid, or totally apathetic. If they possess the natural intelligence and education to understand the information you may try to relay to them, they simply won't care. Faced with this knowledge, why should you invite failure by trying to teach these people how to call for help in a crisis?

The answer is simple, and it rests on your understanding of *who the public is*. The general nameless, faceless public is made up of individuals. Each individual has a life; each works, and eats, and sleeps, and plays. Each one loves, and each one grieves. Each one lives, and every life is important. In choosing medical communication as your profession, you have dedicated your efforts to the preservation of life. *If you can save or positively impact even one life by implementing a public education and information program, you can congratulate yourself on a job well done.*

Educating the Public: When to Try

There are six logical points in the development of an EMS system when your chances of conducting a successful information campaign are better than at other, more "normal" times. They are:

- *During or prior to the start-up of a new system.* Since you are largely an unknown entity to your public, you can literally define your own role in the community. You possess a public relations advantage now that you may never have again; don't waste it!
- *When a major component either changes or is added to your system*; for example, when a 9-1-1 system goes on-line or when your CAD system is upgraded. This can create an interest which will motivate your public to read, listen, and learn.
- *On the anniversary of the item above*, the process may be repeated with good results. Contact a local media representative just before the time when the addition or change has been in place for 1 year, 2 years, or 5 years. Provide the rep with positive examples of how the addition has contributed to good patient care. Create a retrospective account of changes in your system, and then review access methods and types of help that are available (pre-arrival instructions, etc.).
- *During any specially designated time period* which relates to our

---

[1] Susan Flader, *Thinking Like a Mountain*, Columbia: University of Missouri Press, 1974; as quoted by Scott M. Cutlip and Allen H. Center in *Effective Public Relations, 5th Edition*, Prentice-Hall, Inc., 1978.

profession, for example, National Health Care Month or a locally identified EMS Week. The public's attention will already be focused in your direction; take advantage of it.

- *When an incident in another service area is receiving frequent bad press.* Never pass up the opportunity to reassure your public that this type of negative outcome cannot happen in your area. Explain and demonstrate why. This is also a good time to review your procedures and safeguards against error; better make sure your house is clean before you invite the neighbors in.
- *When an incident in your own service area has an exceptionally good outcome.* For example, your system's communicators talk a caller through delivering a baby or performing life-saving CPR. Calls involving children are especially effective. The general public reacts to pediatric calls exactly the way EMS professionals do: there is greater emotional involvement, and the call is remembered longer. It's not only technical excellence that makes a call outstanding; it's also the human element. Don't be afraid to pat yourself on the back when you do your job exceptionally well.

What to Do and How to Do It

How to start? Where to begin? First, devise a plan for your system; write it down. Include a proposed time schedule and commit to meeting your goals, in both the areas of achievement and time. Your plan should include any or all of the following:

- *Identify one person to serve as your system's designated media contact.*
- *Arrange for newspaper, radio, and television investigators and reporters to visit your communications center.* Explain the equipment. Outline for them the educational process for EMS personnel. Allow them to listen while you receive and process calls for help, prioritize the responses, and give pre-arrival instructions. Bring them into your world, and show them how it works.
- *Explain to the media representatives what offends EMS personnel.* Most reporters don't call us *"ambulance drivers"* with the intent to make us angry or to insult us; they have never been told what the terms are which are acceptable to us.
- *Obtain telephone numbers and establish procedures for notifying media personnel when a newsworthy event takes place within your system.* Give media reps appropriate nonemergency numbers to call when they need information. *Each player in the process of information exchange should have knowledge of the constraints under which the other operates.* While EMS personnel expect reporters to understand that medical communicators are busy completing important, life-saving tasks, the courtesy is rarely extended in reverse. When you call a reporter to relay information about an event, it's appropriate to ask right away, "Are you on deadline, or do you have a minute to talk?"

Chap. 15   Public Relations   157

- *Within your organization, train speakers to make public appearances.* Make sure your designated speakers are personable, well-informed, and always dressed in *perfect* uniforms.
- *Devise personal appearance programs that target specific audiences*, such as:

    *Preschool age children.* Provide pictures and line drawings as visual aids. Arrive in an ambulance and let the kids sit in it. Allow them to touch bandaging and splinting supplies; let them bounce on the stretcher. Concentrate on relieving the very young child's fears of injury and the unknown. Explain to the children how to dial 9-1-1; help them to practice on a toy telephone. Assure them that someone just like you will answer the phone when they call, and that whoever answers will help them. Answer questions as honestly as you can without frightening your audience, and leave a printed handout with each child. Handouts should include emergency and nonemergency telephone numbers for your system, and describe the kinds of help that are available. Tell each child to take the printed material home to her or his parents.

    *Elementary school-age children.* Pull equipment off the unit and show them how it works. Take blood pressures, being careful not to pump the the cuff up too tight. Run EKGs on a few of the kids, and give them the strips to take home. Splint an imaginary fractured arm. Place a pretend patient on a backboard and demonstrate proper lifting techniques. Position a child on the stretcher; then raise and lower it, and roll it around. Explain who will answer the phone when your audience calls for help and what kind of information the call-taker will ask for. Stress to the children the importance of not hanging up until they're told to. Tell the group what your local penalties are for making 9-1-1 calls when no real emergency exists. Also, help them understand that fake calls take ambulances away from people who really need help and may die without it. Follow up by making sure they understand that, when in doubt, they should *always* call. Emphasize that you won't be angry with them if they call because they're not sure it's an emergency. Distribute a handout for the kids' parents.

    *Middle and high school groups: adolescents and young adults.* Again, pull out equipment and demonstrate its use. Explain in more detail vital signs, EKGs, oxygen delivery, anti-shock garments, and any medications *except* narcotics. *Never* advertise the fact that you carry narcotics.

    Tell the group "war stories," taking care to maintain patient confidentiality. Ask the students about their experiences in emergency situations and with ambulances. Explain how to access the system. Discuss career opportunities and training requirements. *Take advantage of any and every opportunity to describe the catastrophic results of alcohol and drug abuse.*

    *Senior citizens' groups.* Travel to activity centers, day care centers, retirement residences. Treat your audience with dignity and respect. Explain the various services you can offer. Be prepared to discuss money: your audience will want information about costs, billing, insurance, Medicare, and other health care supplements. *If you are not an expert in the area of billing and insurance, take someone with you who is; you must be very careful not to give your audience incorrect information.* Many systems offer subscription plans at reduced costs for seniors; bring printed material to leave with your audience.

Don't assume that because your listeners are elderly, they are incapacitated and cannot perform life-saving intervention. Describe to them the signs and symptoms of various illnesses and injuries, and appropriate first aid techniques. Encourage both residents and staff to complete CPR training. Remember that the elderly fear illness, injury, financial reverses, death, and loss of control. You can offer them comfort by telling them what to do to regain some of that control in an emergency.

*Professional and church groups.* Offer to take your presentations to meetings of Rotary and Lions Clubs, church groups, women's professional organizations, and the like. Explain the technical innovations in your system, the size and population of your service area, and the number of calls run per year. Describe the educational and quality control processes in place. Briefly explain the principles of system status management. Tell a few "war stories"; balance funny situations with descriptions of negative outcomes that could have been avoided.

If your communications center is not the primary PSAP for your local 9-1-1 system, describe the "dead air" sound that callers hear when a call is transferred. Explain the advantages of medical prioritization and pre-arrival instructions, and provide some examples.

Encourage parents to teach their children how to access the emergency medical response system. Make sure adults understand the importance of placing at least one telephone where even small children can reach it.

With any specific target group, explain to your audience the basics of the hysterical reaction. Provide them with reassurance that the system *will* work for them. Tell your listeners what to expect when they call for help, and emphasize again the importance of medical prioritization and pre-arrival instructions. Remind your audience not to hang up.

## CONTRIBUTING TO CUSTOMER SATISFACTION

Like many medical communicators, I first worked in the field setting. Years ago, when we all worked 24-hour shifts, my home station was located in a section of the city known for its high incidence of violent crime and the poverty of its residents. We ran a great many calls in a large, densely populated government-subsidized housing project. Gradually, I came to know many of the residents in "the project" well.

On summer nights in Texas, the temperature frequently stalls above 90 degrees, even at 10:00 P.M. Late at night, a group of elderly men would gather on a street corner in the project; it was cooler outside than it was in their apartments. Those old men played some of the best guitar and sang some of the best "scat" I've ever heard. Whenever we were awake and in the neighborhood, we would stop by the corner; the old men would usually invite me to play and sing with them. They even brought an extra guitar, in case I showed up. Eventually, I became part of their informal extended family.

Early one morning, my partner and I were called to the residence of one of these old gentlemen, a man named Willie Ray. It was obvious as soon as we walked in the door that Willie Ray was in trouble. He had been recently diagnosed as having end-stage congestive heart failure; now he presented with pulmonary edema. I called for drug orders and did everything the physician and I together could think of, and none of it did any good. Willie was conscious the entire time, and working *so* hard to breathe; I didn't spend much time on the scene. As we began our hospital return, I was still frantically working to reverse Willie's fluid overload. Although I didn't realize it, I guess I was also frowning pretty fiercely as I tried to concentrate, do six things at once, and hold myself together emotionally. I loved that old man, and I hated to see him suffer.

Five minutes away from the hospital, Willie Ray pulled my hair and said, *"You never know when you're making a memory....Give me a smile, girl; I'll be taking it with me as long as I can."* Then he closed his eyes. We delivered him to the emergency department, and when we were called out from the hospital to make another response, he was still alive.

There is no happy ending to this story; Willie Ray didn't survive. I, however, had my superior little attitude changed by a destitute 84-year-old man who never made it past the third grade. I have never forgotten what Willie said. He made me realize that my five-second display of bad temper or inappropriate attitude could, at any time, form the only image of my character and my profession that any observers might take away with them. It only takes a second or two to make an impression, whether good or bad. It's a sobering thought.

Always remember that each person from whom you receive a telephone call, whether for emergency or nonemergency service, to request information or to file a complaint, is a *person*. Each is entitled to your attention and respect.

Stop and review the chapters on Basic Communication and Telecommunication Theory, Advanced Telecommunications Techniques, and The Psychology of Dealing with the Person in Crisis. Now take the time to thoroughly consider this: *There are almost 1,500 minutes in any 24-hour day. Each and every one of those minutes can and will present you with the opportunity to form, change, or confirm a caller's impression or image of you as a medical communicator, your communications department, your system, and our profession as a whole.*

Receiving the respect that you as EMS professionals desire and deserve, and ensuring the continued success of your system depend on your behavior in the communications center *every shift that you work.* You must take advantage of every opportunity to make each contact beneficial and each impression a positive one.

## SUMMARY AND REVIEW

1. Define public relations.

2. What steps are involved in the relay of information?

3. What items of information concerning a patient or a response can safely be released to the media?

4. Why should administrators be notified of major media events?

5. What are some of the most commonly encountered barriers to change?

6. At what points in the development of an EMS system can you predict a favorable response to public relations efforts?

7. Outline for your system a series of steps that make up a plan for public education.

# Chapter 16

# QUALITY ASSURANCE AND QUALITY IMPROVMENT IN EMERGENCY MEDICAL DISPATCHING

*"Take what you want," said God.*
*"Take what you want . . . and then pay for it."*
— *Old Spanish Proverb*

## THE NEED FOR QUALITY ASSURANCE

At one time, we in EMS service considered ourselves to be "a breed apart"; we made our own rules, and functioned, not always successfully, independently from those guidelines that governed standard business practices in other industries. In recent years, interesting developments have occurred in the American marketplace, and particularly among the providers of pre-hospital medical care and transportation.

Today, in the face of increased competition in the marketplace, declining domestic productivity, and a marked increase in participation by foreign investors, American managers in emergency medical service must learn to provide a wider range of services, better quality patient care, and a high level of customer satisfaction. In many areas, the days when one service was "the only game in town" are over. Our customers, whether private citizens, city governments, or government subcontracted administrative agencies, have become better educated and better informed. Our clients now understand that they *do* have choices, and they know how to exercise them. Those officers, administrators, services, and systems who can't or won't "get with the program" will not survive the continuing changes in our industry.

## UTILIZING THE TEAM APPROACH

At one time, the majority of American workers were in manufacturing rather than service. Now the number of service jobs exceeds those in the manufacturing area.

A funny thing happened on the way to the marketplace. As the American consumer "grew up," so did the American worker. As our customers realized that they had choices in what they would allow and expect in terms of service and product delivered, the workers stopped accepting "Because I said so" as a reason for doing anything. EMS workers in particular expect and deserve to be told why a procedure is implemented; they are entitled to become part of the process.

Employee involvement is one approach to improving quality and productivity with cooperative relationships, open communication, and group problem solving and decision making. This approach has received substantial credit for contributing to quality and productivity improvement in a number of countries, most notably Japan. Participation and employee involvement have also been successful in the United States in both manufacturing and service industries.

It is estimated that there are now approximately two hundred thousand employee involvement groups in the United States, and several million operating worldwide.[1]

## QUALITY ASSURANCE IN EMERGENCY MEDICAL SERVICE

While quality assurance is a vital element in any private industry committed to establishing and holding its niche in an increasingly competitive marketplace, the consistent delivery of the highest quality service is absolutely essential for a business such as ours.

If we manufactured tennis shoes and our production quality fell below acceptable industry standards, the worst that could happen is that a customer's tennis shoe might fall apart. While experiencing a high-top blowout when jogging at 5 or 6 miles per hour could certainly be an emotionally traumatic occurrence, the chance of loss of life or permanent disability would be minimal. Since we deal in the care, treatment, and transportation of ill and injured human beings, we must all constantly and aggressively work to keep our incidence of error to an absolute minimum. *Patient care begins the instant that conversation begins with the caller.*

## TYPES OF ERRORS IN THE COMMUNICATIONS CENTER

Errors made in any medical dispatch center may be classified into two broad categories: unavoidable mistakes, and those that, through forethought and planning, may be avoided.

*Unavoidable* errors result from "bad" or incorrect information given by the caller, lack of reliable information (frequently, but not always, from third-party callers), situations not previously experienced, and so on. While a certain number of these errors will always

---

[1] Charles A. Aubrey, II and Patricia K. Felkins, "Teamwork: Involving People in Quality and Productivity Improvement," American Society for Quality Control, 1988.

occur, mistakes can, with effort, be recategorized from unavoidable to avoidable, and then averted altogether.

*Avoidable* errors can and must be prevented from taking place. This goal can be achieved through the establishment of a rigorous set of standards to include strong medical control, standardized algorithms for telephone triage interviewing and remote intervention techniques, standardized position statements and detailed procedures, careful screening and selection of candidates for training as system status controllers, a comprehensive initial training program, regularly scheduled and evaluated written examinations, on-site and on-duty supervisory suggestions for improvement, ongoing training and retraining, continuing education, scheduled performance reviews, clinical information feedback reports, audio tape reviews, and monthly analyses of response time compliance percentages by communicator.

## MEDICAL CONTROL

What, exactly, is medical control? For the purposes of emergency medical dispatching, *medical control is the process of ensuring that actions taken on behalf of ill or injured persons are medically appropriate.* This includes the activities of prioritization of EMS responses and delivery of pre-arrival instructions.[2]

Medical control is accomplished in several phases: First, telephone triage and remote intervention instructions are initially written, reviewed, and approved by the communications administrator, the system clinical coordinator, the physician medical director, and the physicians' advisory group. These standardized formats should be reviewed annually (or more frequently) by selected medical dispatchers, the communications manager, and the clinical coordinator. When this review process is complete, suggestions for changes, refinements, and improvements should be presented to the physicians' advisory group for approval. These changes must reflect similar changes in locally and nationally utilized standards.

Second, a thoroughly researched and detailed system of candidate selection, training, retraining, written testing, and timed performance evaluations must be established and all participants must comply with established standards.

Third, the communications division as a department should be allowed and encouraged to establish its own performance standards which meet or exceed any standard imposed by any governmental or contractual requirement. In some systems, a self-policing committee of line communicators can perform routine performance audits to monitor dispatchers' adherence to approved guidelines. In other EMS response systems, outside evaluation may be necessary. In addition to routine compliance with established performance standards, other specific types of incidents should be reviewed, that is, "problem" calls;

---

[2] Clawson and Dernocoeur, EMT-P, "Principles of Emergency Medical Dispatch," p. 239.

responses where the hospital return is run at a more critical priority than that at which the call was dispatched; multiple unit responses, and so on. These audits should be routinely conducted jointly by the medical dispatchers involved, the communicators' tape review committee, the communications administrator, and the clinical coordinator; paramedic operations supervisors, field crew members, a field run review committee, the system medical director, and/or the chief executive officer should participate as appropriate. Selected cases may then be submitted for review to the physicians' advisory group at the joint direction of the communications administrator and the clinical coordinator.

In any medically sound system, the clinical coordinator must be acknowledged as the first avenue of medical review outside the department for the medical communicator; frequent, open communication between the medical dispatcher and the clinical coordinator should be strongly encouraged.

## STANDARDIZATION OF TELEPHONE PROCEDURES

*"The protruding nail gets hammered."*
*— Buddhist proverb*

Standardized algorithms for telephone triage and remote intervention instructions are utilized in progressive communications systems for two reasons: They provide protection for the patient, and they provide protection for the care-giver, in this case the medical communicator. The basic concepts and practicality involved in using these algorithms have been tried and tested in systems nationwide, and have been proven medically and legally sound. To be safe and effective, medically approved algorithms must be followed *exactly and completely* during the processing of *each and every* call for help.

*If the algorithms are followed, your patient will be assured of the optimum in care, and, based on current test case decisions, you will be protected against personal liability in case of litigation. If you do not follow the protocols, it will be because you have made a conscious, deliberate choice not to do so. If you choose not to follow your system's established protocols and your actions are later questioned or criticized, you will probably find that you stand on your own. Legal advisors and advocates for you, your department, and your system will be unable to maximize their abilities to defend you, because you will have acted outside established guidelines.*

## POSITION STATEMENTS AND PROCEDURES

The command structure or management staff of every system should provide to the medical communicator both broad-based position statements and detailed policies and procedures governing every aspect of the dispatcher's job. The general intent contained in the position statements, combined with specific procedural instructions, should serve to direct the actions of the dispatcher in almost every eventuality and type of incident occurrence. In any situation for which specific procedures have not been standardized, the *general intent* of established position statements should be clear enough to be easily followed, and the communications manager or other administrator should be contacted for advice and direction. *Patient care, crew safety, and intelligent allocation of resources must always remain top priorities.*

## CANDIDATE SELECTION

The most commonly overlooked opportunity to affect the overall quality of work produced in any communications center lies in the initial selection of candidates or applicants to train for a dispatcher's position. There have traditionally been no widely recognized and accepted methods to measure a potential candidate's aptitude for the job. In many systems, assignment to the communications department has been used as a punishment when an employee's field performance becomes unacceptable. In others, field employees who have exhibited signs of field stress overload, or who have been physically injured on the job, are temporarily assigned to the control center for "light duty." *This position has become much too critical to allow its use as a "dumping ground."* If an employee cannot, due to stress or disciplinary problems, meet the criteria for one department in a system, she/he *must not* be casually transferred to another department. It must also never be assumed that, because an injured field care-giver performed her/his field job satisfactorily, she/he is capable of performing the medical communicator's job equally well. We should never simply relocate a problem; we should identify it and resolve it. Retrain the employee, re-evaluate the employee, mandate the employee into professional counseling, but *do not* re-assign the problem employee to a crucially important department whose employees are at the highest risk for critical error and litigation.

## SETTING MINIMUM PREREQUISITE STANDARDS

Strict standards and prerequisites for the medical communicator's position must be established, *and our hiring practices must reflect a faithful compliance to those standards.* Prerequisites will vary according to the needs of different systems. These are some suggestions for basic requirements that must be satisfied before a candidate is accepted into the application process for the medical communicator's position:

- Set a minimum standard for the level of *medical training* achieved. Two schools of thought exist as to what that standard should be. Although nonmedical personnel are routinely and successfully trained to perform this job, training time is frequently shorter and end job performance is, in some cases, of higher quality when medical training has already been accomplished. However, advanced medical training may, on occasion, become an actual drawback; when not enough structure is provided, dispatchers with extensive medical knowledge or field experience sometimes decide that they are smarter than the protocols. Your system may require certification to the basic emergency medical technician level, or you may require paramedic-level training. Nursing personnel may also be employed successfully, provided they are cross-trained and certified to work on an ambulance, or some other mechanism (field ride-outs, for example) is provided to help them gain a working knowledge of the field aspect of the emergency medical response system.

- It is strongly recommended that a minimum *experience level* be set. A usable working knowledge of EMS systems today includes such elements as knowledge of the range of services available, first responder and mutual aid capabilities, field medical protocols, relays of patient information to base hospitals, procedures for ancillary personnel, trouble-shooting and repairing both communications and field equipment. The medical communicator today must be able to function in a supervisory capacity when required. It is impossible to accomplish this without a complete working knowledge of the system itself. Candidates with a minimum of 6 months *working experience* in a system will usually require less training time and may have higher skills levels and better chances for ultimate success than those with no system experience.

- In order to effectively learn the use of intervention techniques, it is strongly recommended that each applicant be *currently certified to provide CPR*.

## THE SELECTION PROCESS

First, the communications department and management must know *when and how* personnel will be recruited and selected to train for communications positions. Planning ahead can and will dramatically reduce short-notice scheduling crises. Rather than waiting until a medical dispatcher leaves the job unexpectedly, *project your department's upcoming personnel needs*.

To ensure that your division's application and selection process is fair and equitable, you must set guidelines for when you will train new communicators. For example, your needs may dictate that you identify qualified training prospects only once or twice yearly. In high volume communications systems with high turnover rates, the training process may be continuous.

When a training position becomes available, notice should be posted of opportunities to enter the program. Notification should be advertised in any forum where it may be available to prospective candidates for employment. If advancement to the communications department is an option for your system's field employees, notification should also be made directly and in writing to each employee in the system via the postal service, voice mail, or interoffice mail. Additional notices should be posted in areas that might be commonly accessed by interested and qualified persons (meeting rooms, field crews' quarters, hospital bulletin boards, etc.). A schedule of dates for interviews and testing should be listed. Set a standard for how much time will elapse between when the notification is posted and when the interviews and testing will take place; then stick to the standard each time you go through the hiring procedure. To allow interested parties reasonable access to the hiring procedure, the first of the posted dates for interviews and testing should be not less than 14 days after the notice is issued. Interested parties should be instructed to contact a specific person or position within the system to arrange dates and times for application interviews and for the administration of written tests. After scheduling is complete, a follow-up call should be made to each applicant, confirming her/his date and time to be interviewed and tested.

An initial interview should be conducted with each applicant, either by the communications supervisor or manager or by an interview board comprised of medical dispatchers, the communications department manager, and other administrative personnel. Each applicant must be asked *standardized* questions, the answers to which have pre-assigned point values. An objective scoring method must be established *before* the interview takes place, and *the same method must be used during each candidate's application process.*

The method used to evaluate the desirability of the applicant should measure ability in two areas. The first is a broad category that summarizes the applicant's attitudes, orientation, and self-knowledge. The second evaluates the candidate's specific availability to fulfill the scheduling needs of the department.

In any communications system, the applicant's ability to fulfill specific scheduling needs must be addressed during the interview process (see Figure 16.1). Points earned are noted on these standardized forms during each interview. The personnel in each system must define their own information-gathering and measurement processes, and should be aware that adjustments must be made as system and department needs change.

While the interviewers are entitled to assess the *measurement* of each applicant's in-place time commitments and her/his time availability to train and to work as a communicator, *questions about the candidate's personal lives must be carefully avoided.* When you have completed what you believe is a workable format to "score" an applicant during an interview, have the form reviewed for content by your system's EEOC representative.

In any system, the information gathered from each candidate should include:

- Length of time employed in the system

| | |
|---|---|
| Medical Dispatch Training Candidate Name: | Date: |
| 1. What is your certification level? | (Info only; No point score) |
| How many years since your original certification? | |
| 0-1 year = 2 points; 1.1-2 years = 4 points; 2.1-3 years = 6 points; | |
| 3.1-4 years = 8 points; 4.1-5 years = 10 points; 5+ years = 15 points. | |
| Points Possible = 15 | Points Earned = |
| 2. How long have you been employed in this system? | |
| 0-1 year = 2 points; 1.1-2 years = 5 points; 2.1-3 years = 10 points; | |
| 3+ years = 15 points. | |
| Points Possible = 15 | Points Earned = |
| 3. Have you worked for another medical transport service in or adjacent to this service area? | No = 0 points; Yes = 5 points |
| Points Possible = 5 | Points Earned = |

4. What shift days and hours do you work in the field?

| Sunday | Monday | Tuesday | Wednesday | Thursday | Friday | Saturday |
|---|---|---|---|---|---|---|
| | | | | | | |

| | |
|---|---|
| Is Saturday am or pm available without field time scheduled for the period of 12 hours before and after? | Yes = 10 points; No = 0 points. |
| Is Sunday am or pm available without field time scheduled for the period of 12 hours before and after? | Yes = 10 points; No = 0 points. |
| Do you work a 24-hour field shift? | Yes = 10 points; No = 0 points. |
| Do you work a 12-hour field shift? | Yes = 5 points; No = 0 points. |
| Do you work a 9-hour field shift? | Yes = 0 points; No = 0 points. |
| Points Possible = 30 | Points Earned = |
| 5. Is your field shift considered a permanent assignment? | |
| | Yes = 5 points; No = 0 points. |
| Points Possible = 5 | Points Earned = |
| Page 1 Total Points Possible = 70 | Page 1 Total Points Earned = |

Figure 16.1 *Interview evaluation forms*

| |
|---|
| Medical Dispatch Training Candidate Name:                         Date: |
| 6. What date were you released to work as a primary field care-giver in this system?  Compute years since released. |
| 0-1 year = 5 points;  1.1-2 years = 10 points;  2.1-3 years = 15 points; 3+ years = 20 points. |
| Points Possible = 20                                    Points Earned = |
| 7. How long have you lived in this service area?  Not living within service area = 0 points;  0-2 years = 5 points; 2.1-3 years = 10 points; 3.1-5 years = 15 points; 5+ years = 20 points. |
| Points Possible = 20                                    Points Earned = |
| 8. Aside from your field shifts, in what other system-related activvities do you participate?  ACLS instructor? If yes, -5 points; field preceptor? If yes, +5 points; field training officer?  If yes, -5 points;  PHTLS faculty?  If yes, -5 points;  CPR instructor?  If yes, +5 points. Are you basic CPR certified?  If yes, +10 points. |
| Points Possible = 20                                    Points Earned = |
| 9. Have you ever worked as a dispatcher?  Yes = 10 points; No = 0 points. |
| Points Possible = 10                                    Points Earned = |
| 10. If the answer to 9 is yes, was your experience with an emergency public service agency?  Yes = 10 points; No = 0 points. |
| Points Possible = 10                                    Points Earned = |
| 11. If the answer to 9 is yes, was your experience with an ambulance service?  Yes = 10 points; No = 0 points. |
| Points Possible = 10                                    Points Earned = |
| 12. If the answer to 9 is yes, did you work with a computer assisted dispatch system?  Yes = 10 points; No = 0 points. |
| Points Possible = 10                                    Points Earned = |
| Page 2 Total Points Possible = 100     Page 2 Total Points Earned = |

Figure 16.1  (continued)

| | |
|---|---|
| Medical Dispatch Training Candidate Name: | Date: |
| 13. Have you ever worked with a personal computer? Yes = 15 points. | |
| Points Possible = 15 | Points Earned = |
| 14. If the answer to 13 is yes, what programs can you efficiently use?  Lotus = 10 points; Q & A = 10 points; DbaseIV = 10 points. | |
| Points Possible = 30 | Points Earned = |
| 15. Do you own a personal computer? Yes = 10 points; No = 0 points. | |
| Points Possible = 10 | Points Earned = |
| 16. Define system status management. | |
| "Making the most efficient use of available resources." = 20 points. | |
| "Positioning units where the next call will come in." = 10 points. | |
| Other answers = 0 points. | |
| Points Possible = 30 | Points Earned = |
| 17. What is the primary job of the medical communicator? | |
| "Ensure the highest quality patient care." = 25 points.  "Getting the care-givers to the patient in the appropriate time." = 15 points. | |
| "Communication." = 10 points. | |
| Points Possible = 50 | Points Earned = |
| 18. In the field setting, what is your favorite type of call? | |
| Trauma = 0 points;  Non-emergency transport = 5 points; Pediatric = 10 points; Major medicine = 15 points. | |
| Points Possible = 15 | Points Earned = |
| 19. What kind of call bothers you the most? Non-emergency transport = -10 points; Major medicine = -5 points;  all others, 0 points. | |
| Points Possible = -10 | Points Earned = |
| 20. Are you seeking a full-time communicator position? Yes = 25 points. Part-time? Yes = 15 points. | |
| Points Possible = 25 | Points Earned = |
| Page 3 Total Points Possible = 165 | Page 3 Total Points Earned = |

Figure 16.1 *(continued)*

| |
|---|
| Medical Dispatch Training Candidate Name:          Date: |
| 21. What is your greatest strength as a care-giver? Any technical skill identified = 0 points; any "people" skill (understanding, compassion, scene management, etc.) = 10 points. Use only first skill identified. |
| Points Possible = 10                                              Points Earned = |
| 22. What is your greatest weakness as a care-giver? Any technical skill identified = 0 points; any "people" skill = -10 points. |
| Points Possible = 0                                               Points Earned = |
| 23. What things make you feel stressed? Specific factors immediately verbalized? Yes = 15 points; No = -15 points. Note factors identified (no assigned point value). |
| Points Possible = 15                                              Points Earned = |
| 24. How do you manage your own stress? Specific methods immediately verbalized? Yes = 15 points; No = -15 points. Note methods identified (no assigned point value). |
| Points Possible = 15                                              Points Earned = |
| 25. When you encounter a problem with a field partner, how do you resolve it? "Deal directly with partner" = 15 points; "Consult supervisor" = 5 points; both = 20 points. Any other answer = 0 points. |
| Points Possible = 20                                              Points Earned = |
| 26. How many hours per week or month do you have regularly scheduled time commitments? (Identify number of hours only; do not relate nature of time commitments.) Examples: college classes, firm church commitments, scouting activities, etc. 0-10 hours per month = 10 points; 11-20 hours per month = -10 points; 21+ hours per month = -20 points. |
| Points Possible = 10                                              Points Earned = |
| Page 4 Total Points Possible = 70          Page 3 Total Points Earned = |

Figure 16.1   *(continued)*

| |
|---|
| Medical Dispatch Training Candidate Name:                Date: |
| 27. How many hours a week are you prepared to commit to training? |
| 0-12 = 0 points;   12.1-24 = 10 points;   24.1-36 = 20 points. |
| Points Possible = 20                                    Points Earned = |
| 28. How much notice do you require to be able to work a voluntary overtime shift?   <12 hours = 10 points; 12-24 hours = 5 points; 24+ hours = 0 points. |
| Points Possible = 10                                    Points Earned = |
| 29. If called in to work a shift in the communications center on an emergency basis, how long would it take you to arrive at the dispatch center?  Count preparation time plus travel time.  <30 minutes = 10 points;  30-60 minutes = 5 points;  60+ minutes = 0 points. |
| Points Possible = 10                                    Points Earned = |
| 30. Can you type?  Yes = 10 points;  No = -10 points. |
| Points Possible = 10                                    Points Earned = |
| 31. If the answer to 30 is yes, how many words per minute can you type? 0-20 = 0 points;  21-40 = 10 points;  41+ = 15 points.  Add points only if actual score on typing test meets or exceeds this estimate. |
| Points Possible = 15                                    Points Earned = |
| 32. Why do you want to train and work as a medical communicator? "Broad perspective" = 10 points;  "Gain knowledge" = 10 points; "Natural progression" = 10 points. |
| Points Possible = 30                                    Points Earned = |
| 33. We utilize a communicator call-back system under which each full-time dispatcher signs up for 2 24-hour call-back periods each month; each alternate dispatcher signs up for 1 shift. Would you agree to participate in this program?  Yes = 20 points;  No = 0 points. |
| Points Possible = 20                                    Points Earned = |
| Page 5 Total Points Possible = 115      Page 5 Total Points Earned = |

Figure 16.1   (continued)

| | |
|---|---|
| Medical Dispatch Training Candidate Name: | Date: |
| 34. Did candidate reschedule date and time of interview more than once? Yes = -10 points. ||
| Points Possible = -10 | Points Earned = |
| 35. Was the candidate tardy for this interview? Yes = -10 points. ||
| Points Possible = -10 | Points Earned = |
| Page 6 Total Points Possible = -20 | Page 6 Total Points Earned = |

| Interview Summary | Points Possible | Points Earned | Percentage |
|---|---|---|---|
| Page 1 | 70 | | |
| Page 2 | 100 | | |
| Page 3 | 165 | | |
| Page 4 | 70 | | |
| Page 5 | 115 | | |
| Page 6 | -20 | | |
| Total All Pages | 500 | | |

Persons present during interview:

### Summary of Application Process

| Section or Event | Date or Interval | Points Possible | Points Earned | Percentage Accurate |
|---|---|---|---|---|
| Oral Interview | | 500 | | |
| Level 1 Written Exam | | 500 | | |
| Typing Test | | 100 | | |
| Work History | | | | |
| Total All Sections | | | | |

### Comparison of Total Scores in Applicant Group

| | |
|---|---|
| | |
| | |
| | |
| | |

Figure 16.1 *(continued)*

- Length of time worked at current certification level
- Present position
- Time in present position
- Whether applicant desires a full-time or alternate (part-time) communicator's position
- Days and hours of current field shift assignment
- Hours per week (not nature) of time commitments and obligations away from the system
- Number of hours weekly the candidate is available to train
- Estimated travel time to the communications center if called in on an emergency basis
- The candidate's perception of the duties of the medical communicator
- The candidate's perception of primary stress factors, generalized for field personnel and personalized
- The candidate's methods of dealing with personal stress and evaluation of her/his success rate in dealing with personal stress
- Candidate's reasons for wanting to train as a medical dispatcher
- Candidate's evaluation of her/his own ability to work as a team member and elicit cooperative attitudes from co-workers

Each candidate must be given the opportunity to ask questions and make whatever statements she/he desires.

When employees are requesting to transfer from field operations to the communications division, information on candidates' work records, disciplinary histories, and documented strengths and weaknesses should be obtained from field operations supervisors by the communications administrator or manager (see Figure 16.2). This information must be held in strictest confidence, and discussed only among managers or supervisors. Input should also be solicited from the clinical coordinator, the operations manager, the chief executive officer, and field training officers, as appropriate.

## CANDIDATE TESTING

If a CAD system is in place in the communications center, a standardized typing test should be administered. Computer programs that are accessible from a stand-alone personal computer and that both teach and evaluate typing skills are readily available at minimal cost. Applicants should also be required to take an entry level (Level 1) general knowledge written examination with a possible score of not less than 500 points. Scores from all four parts of the process (interviews, work histories, typing tests, and written examinations) should be computed. Applicants should be notified, preferably in writing, of the outcome of the testing and evaluation process. Scores should be listed from highest point score to lowest, and applicants accepted into training positions based on those scores.

| INTERDEPARTMENTAL REQUEST FOR WORK HISTORY INFORMATION |||||||
|---|---|---|---|---|---|---|
| From | | Title | | Department ||||
| To | | Title | | Department ||||
| , currently employed in your department, has asked to be considered for a training position in Medical Communications. Please complete and return this request at your earliest convenience. |||||||
| Employee Date of Birth || Date of Hire ||| SSN ||
| Current position |||||| Annual salary |
| Performance Appraisal History |||||||
| Date | By | Type (60 day, 90 day, etc. | Pts Avail/ Pts Earned | S/U | # Shifts Sched | Attendance/ Punctuality | Comms Use |
| | | | | | | | |
| | | | | | | | |
| | | | | | | | |
| | | | | | | | |
| | | | | | | | |
| Record of Commendations |||||||
| Date | By | Action/Comments ||||| Comms Use |
| | | | | | | | |
| | | | | | | | |
| | | | | | | | |
| Record of Disciplinary Action |||||||
| Date | By | Type (Verbal, Written, Susp) || Nature of Problem/ Policy Violated ||| Comms Use |
| | | | | | | | |
| | | | | | | | |
| | | | | | | | |
| Info Completed By |||||| Date |
| Return Date ||| Rec'd By ||| Date |

Figure 16.2 *Interdepartmental request for work history information*

When a training position becomes available in the dispatch center, applicants for the position must be re-evaluated to confirm that the desire to train still exists, and to determine the current compatibility of candidates' time availability and field schedules with the training position schedule. Seniority and work records should again be considered. If two or more candidates are equally qualified for the position, additional standardized testing should be administered to evaluate the candidates' geographic knowledge of the service area, medical protocols, procedures, reactions to situational exercises, and so on. Results of these tests should be used to identify the candidate best qualified for the position.

## THE INITIAL TRAINING PROCESS

*Training as an emergency medical communicator is a process, not an event.* The initial training process should include observation and practice in basic communications and telecommunications theory and techniques, advanced telecommunications techniques, motivation and attitudes, evaluation of typing skills and drills to improve them, written examinations, familiarization with general position statements and specific procedures, documentation and reporting techniques, system status management, and both off-line and on-line, hands-on experience in performing the relay of medical information, nonemergency call-taking, emergency call-taking, telephone triage and interviewing methods, the administration of remote intervention instructions, radio operation, and resource allocation. Each trainee should complete training shifts during day and night hours, and with two or more designated communications trainers.

Remember that your department's communicators must not only be capable of performing their assigned duties, they must be able to prove they can do so. Part of this proof consists of documentation of the initial training process. Hours spent training in each position or in each procedure must be recorded in some type of training documentation package (Figure 16.3). Each communications trainer should complete and supply to the communications manager or communications center training officer written interim evaluations (Figure 16.4) of the trainee's progress, strengths, and weaknesses at two-week intervals throughout the training process. Each of these interim evaluations should then be discussed in depth with the trainee.

When adequate time to ensure acceptable performance in each position and each procedure is complete, and positive evaluations have been received for the same, the trainee enters the final evaluation phase. Each trainee should earn a passing score on a Level 2 medical dispatcher written examination. Typing skills should also be re-evaluated. Finally, each trainee must successfully complete a specified number of final evaluation shifts with the communications director or training coordinator (a minimum of two 12-hour shifts is suggested). Upon successful completion of the final evaluation shifts, the trainee will have concluded the initial training process, and can be released to work as a primary medical communicator.

Chap. 16   *Quality Assurance and Quality Improvement in Emergency Medical Dispatching*   **177**

```
┌─────────────────────────────────────────────────────────────────┐
│           Medical Communicator Training Progress Record         │
├─────────────────────────────────────────────────────────────────┤
│ General Instructions:  Keep the pages in this packet together;  │
│ bring them with you each time you report for a training shift.  │
│ At the end of each training shift, have your trainer initial    │
│ and date each block that applies.                               │
├─────────────────────────────────────────────────────────────────┤
│ Section 1: Information.   Trainee Name:                         │
├─────────────────────────────────────────────────────────────────┤
│ Interview Date:      Typing Test Date:     Written Exam Date:   │
├─────────────────────────────────────────────────────────────────┤
│ On-Site Training Start Date:                                    │
├─────────────────────────────────────────────────────────────────┤
│ Section 2: Training Schedule.  Begin the calendar on the date   │
│ that your first training shift is scheduled (On-Site Training   │
│ Start Date).  Note on each day the hours you worked.  An        │
│ additional calendar is attached; more calendar sheets are       │
│ available when these are complete.                              │
└─────────────────────────────────────────────────────────────────┘
```

| Sun | Mon | Tue | Wed | Thu | Fri | Sat |
|-----|-----|-----|-----|-----|-----|-----|
|     |     |     |     |     |     |     |
|     |     |     |     |     |     |     |
|     |     |     |     |     |     |     |
|     |     |     |     |     |     |     |
|     |     |     |     |     |     |     |
|     |     |     |     |     |     |     |
|     |     |     |     |     |     |     |

Figure 16.3   *Training documentation package*

| Sun | Mon | Tue | Wed | Thu | Fri | Sat |
|-----|-----|-----|-----|-----|-----|-----|
|     |     |     |     |     |     |     |
|     |     |     |     |     |     |     |
|     |     |     |     |     |     |     |
|     |     |     |     |     |     |     |
|     |     |     |     |     |     |     |
|     |     |     |     |     |     |     |
|     |     |     |     |     |     |     |
|     |     |     |     |     |     |     |

Medical Communications Training Schedule
Trainee Name: _____

Figure 16.3  *(continued)*

| Medical Communicator Training Progress Record |||||||
|---|---|---|---|---|---|---|
| Section 3: Procedures. Have your trainer date and initial each task category each shift that you spend time on a particular procedure. ||||||||
| Task or Procedure | Date Performed/Trainer Initials |||||
| 1. Received copy of training manual | | | | | |
| 2. General orientation; physical layout; discussion of manual contents; attitude and motivation explained; "house rules" explained. Performed by communications administrator or assistant. | | | | | |
| 3. Observes medical relay procedure | | | | | |
| 4. Performs medical relay supervised | | | | | |
| 5. Performs medical relay unsupervised | | | | | |
| 6. Observes hospital divert procedures and charting | | | | | |
| 7. Performs hospital divert procedures and charting supervised | | | | | |
| 8. Performs hospital divert procedures and charting unsupervised | | | | | |
| 9. Observes non-emergency call-taking procedures | | | | | |
| 10. Takes non-emergency calls supervised | | | | | |
| 11. Takes non-emergency calls unsupervised | | | | | |
| 12. Observes emergency call-taking procedures | | | | | |
| 13. Takes emergency calls supervised | | | | | |
| 14. Takes emergency calls unsupervised | | | | | |
| 15. Observes radio operator; pre-alerting, dispatching and post move-ups demonstrated/explained | | | | | |
| 16. Acts as radio operator; pre-alerts units, dispatches calls, makes post move-ups supervised | | | | | |
| 17. Acts as radio operator; pre-alerts units, dispatches calls, makes post move-ups unsupervised | | | | | |

Figure 16.3 *(continued)*

| Medical Communicator Training Progress Record ||||||
|---|---|---|---|---|---|
| Section 3: Procedures continued. ||||||
| Task or Procedure | Date Performed/Trainer Initials |||||
| 18. Procedures for documentation and completing paperwork reviewed | | | | | |
| 19. Verifies data in every field of run forms/cards | | | | | |
| 20. Completes response time exception reports, supervised | | | | | |
| 21. Completes response time exception reports, unsupervised | | | | | |
| 22. Computer data entry procedures observed | | | | | |
| 23. Computer data entry performed supervised | | | | | |
| 24. Computer data entry performed unsupervised | | | | | |
| 25. "CAD down" procedures explained | | | | | |
| 26. "CAD down" procedures performed supervised | | | | | |
| 27. "CAD down" procedures performed unsupervised | | | | | |
| 28. Typing test administered (note date and words per minute) | | | | | |
| 29. Assists in keeping work area clean | | | | | |
| 30. System status management and post move-ups discussed in depth as system changes | | | | | |
| 31. Handles administrative traffic supervised | | | | | |
| 32. Handles administrative traffic unsupervised | | | | | |
| 33. Other: | | | | | |
| | | | | | |
| | | | | | |
| | | | | | |
| | | | | | |

Figure 16.3 *(continued)*

| Medical Communicator Training Progress Record |||||||||
|---|---|---|---|---|---|---|---|---|
| Section 4: Evaluation Schedule. Performance evaluations will be performed for the trainee every two weeks, beginning from the on-site training start date. Have your evaluation forms completed by your trainer as close to the scheduled date as possible. Completed evaluation forms will be received by the communications administrator, who will discuss each evaluation with the trainee. |||||||||
| Date Due | Date Performed | Performed By | Points Avail | Points Earned | Pass/ Fail | Rec'd By Admin | Reviewed w/Trainee | Initials Both |
|  |  |  |  |  |  |  |  |  |
|  |  |  |  |  |  |  |  |  |
|  |  |  |  |  |  |  |  |  |
|  |  |  |  |  |  |  |  |  |
|  |  |  |  |  |  |  |  |  |
|  |  |  |  |  |  |  |  |  |
|  |  |  |  |  |  |  |  |  |
|  |  |  |  |  |  |  |  |  |
|  |  |  |  |  |  |  |  |  |
|  |  |  |  |  |  |  |  |  |
|  |  |  |  |  |  |  |  |  |
|  |  |  |  |  |  |  |  |  |
|  |  |  |  |  |  |  |  |  |
|  |  |  |  |  |  |  |  |  |
|  |  |  |  |  |  |  |  |  |
|  |  |  |  |  |  |  |  |  |
|  |  |  |  |  |  |  |  |  |
|  |  |  |  |  |  |  |  |  |
|  |  |  |  |  |  |  |  |  |
|  |  |  |  |  |  |  |  |  |
|  |  |  |  |  |  |  |  |  |
|  |  |  |  |  |  |  |  |  |

Figure 16.3   *(continued)*

| Medical Communicator Training Progress Record |||||||
|---|---|---|---|---|---|---|
| Section 5: Level 2 Testing. |||||||
| Evaluation Tool | Date | Points Avail | Points Earned | % | Pass/ Fail ||
| Typing Test (Note WPM) | | | | | ||
| Level 2 Written Examination | | | | | ||
| Evaluation Shift 1: Radio Operator | | | | | ||
| Non-Emergency Call-Taker | | | | | ||
| Emergency Call-Taker | | | | | ||
| Evaluation Shift 2: Radio Operator | | | | | ||
| Non-Emergency Call-Taker | | | | | ||
| Emergency Call-Taker | | | | | ||
| Summary | | | | | ||

Section 6: Final Recommendations.

Recommendation: That trainee/employee repeat all or part of training process made by:                    Date:

Comments:

Recommendation: That trainee/employee be released into primary medical communicator position made by:                    Date:

Comments:

Shift Assignment:

First Regularly Assigned Shift Worked as Primary:

Next Performance Evaluation Due:

Comments:

Figure 16.3   *(continued)*

Chap. 16  *Quality Assurance and Quality Improvement in Emergency Medical Dispatching*  **183**

| Medical Communicator Performance Evaluation: Emergency Call-Taker |||||
|---|---|---|---|---|
| Employee/Trainee Name: *John Anderson*  Date: *3/12* |||||
| Standard | Yes/No | Points Avail | Points Earned ||
| Answers telephone in 2 rings or less | Yes | 10 | 10 ||
| Answers telephone using standardized phrasing | Yes | 10 | 10 ||
| Verbally obtains/confirms address and call-back number within 15 seconds | sometimes | 15 | 10 ||
| Obtains apartment complex name, bldg no., apt no., business name, entrance, and/or any other info | sometimes | 10 | 7 ||
| Determines problem | Yes | 10 | 10 ||
| Accurately prioritizes call using protocols | Yes | 20 | 20 ||
| Reassures caller: "Help is on the way" | Yes | 15 | 15 ||
| Gives remote intervention instructions as necessary using standardized protocols | Yes | 20 | 20 ||
| Understands and retains information the first time; does not ask caller to repeat | Yes | 10 | 10 ||
| Is easily understood by caller; avoids long silences | silences | 10 | 5 ||
| Uses standardized formats/calming techniques during interrogation to gain constructive control of the conversation | Yes | 10 | 10 ||
| Inspires caller to have confidence in her/his abilities and competence | Yes | 10 | 10 ||
| Completes call-taking process quickly | Yes | 10 | 10 ||
| Promptly notifies appropriate first responders and/or law enforcement personnel | Consistently forgets | 10 | 0 ||
| Displays calm, courteous, professional, caring supportive telephone manner | Yes | 20 | 20 ||
| Demonstrates proficient voice control; uses even, well-modulated, non-irritating tone | Yes | 30 | 30 ||
| Monitors unit status changes; assists radio operator | Yes | 20 | 20 ||
| Completes fair share of work load; prevents personal telephone calls from interfering with performance of job duties | Yes | 20 | 20 ||
| Total Points |  | 260 | 237 ||
| 90% (Passing) = 234 points; 95% (Superior) = 247 points. |||||
| Trainer/Evaluator *Janet Jones*   Reviewed by *S. Smith* |||||

Figure 16.4  *Interim evaluation forms*

| Medical Communicator Performance Evaluation: Radio Operator | | | |
|---|---|---|---|
| Employee/Trainee Name: *John Anderson*    Date: *3/14* | | | |
| Standard | Yes/No | Points Avail | Points Earned |
| Answers field units promptly (within 5 seconds) | yes | 15 | 15 |
| Displays calm, courteous, professional radio manner | yes | 20 | 20 |
| Speaks slowly and clearly | yes | 15 | 15 |
| Pre-alerts closest appropriate unit for each emergency response | some | 15 | 10 |
| Uses approved standardized voice format for pre-alerting and paging units | yes | 15 | 15 |
| Uses approved standardized voice format for dispatching each response | yes | 20 | 20 |
| Includes specific information: type of call, builing name/number, apt number, entrance, business name, routing instructions, scene hazards, etc. | yes | 20 | 20 |
| Makes post move-ups immediately: in 15 seconds or less from each pre-alert and/or dispatch | some | 20 | 15 |
| Gives time EVERY time when acknowledging unit status changes | yes | 15 | 15 |
| Dispatches every call in 60 seconds or less | yes | 15 | 15 |
| Demonstrates proficient voice control; uses even, well-modulated, non-irritating tone | yes | 30 | 30 |
| Constantly monitors unit status changes | some | 20 | 15 |
| Records destination/transport priority on each call | some | 20 | 15 |
| Follows unit deployment plan | yes | 20 | 20 |
| Completes fair share of work load; prevents personal telephone calls from interfering with performance of job duties | yes | 20 | 20 |
| Total Points | | 280 | 260 |
| 90% (Passing) = 252 points; 95% (Superior) = 266 points. | | | |
| Trainer/Evaluator *Janet Jones*    Reviewed by *S. Smith* | | | |

Figure 16.4 *(continued)*

| Medical Communicator Performance Evaluation: Non-Emergency Call-Taker |||||
|---|---|---|---|---|
| Employee/Trainee Name: *John Anderson* | | Date: *3/15* |||
| Standard | | Yes/No | Points Avail | Points Earned |
| Answers telephone in 2 rings or less | | yes | 10 | 10 |
| Answers telephone using standardized phrasing | | yes | 10 | 10 |
| Obtains calling party's name and call-back number | | yes | 10 | 10 |
| Obtains address/facility name, hall, station, room, department, patient name, destination address, appointment time/nature, and/or any other info | | yes | 20 | 20 |
| Determines problem | | yes | 10 | 10 |
| Accurately prioritizes call using protocols | | yes | 20 | 20 |
| Checks number of previously scheduled calls/hour | | yes | 15 | 15 |
| Negotiates acceptable pickup time with caller | | yes | 20 | 20 |
| Understands and retains information the first time; does not ask caller to repeat | | yes | 10 | 10 |
| Is easily understood by caller; avoids long silences | | yes | 10 | 10 |
| Handles complaint calls calmly; attempts to identify the nature of the problem/department to contact; accurately records name/number to return call | | argued caller | 10 | 0 |
| Inspires caller to have confidence in her/his abilities and competence | | yes | 10 | 10 |
| Enters call information quickly/accurately *call entry still slow* | | | 10 | 5 |
| Promptly notifies personnel of emergency messages | | yes | 10 | 10 |
| Displays calm, courteous, professional, caring supportive telephone manner | | yes | 20 | 20 |
| Demonstrates proficient voice control; uses even, well-modulated, non-irritating tone | | yes | 30 | 30 |
| Monitors unit status changes; assists radio operator | | yes | 20 | 20 |
| Completes fair share of work load; prevents personal telephone calls from interfering with performance of job duties | | yes | 20 | 20 |
| Total Points | | | 265 | 250 |
| 90% (Passing) = 238 points; 95% (Superior) = 252 points. |||||
| Trainer/Evaluator *Janet Jones* | | Reviewed by *S. Smith* |||

Figure 16.4 *(continued)*

## INTERIM PERFORMANCE APPRAISALS

Routine audio tape reviews and interim performance evaluations should be conducted throughout each ensuing evaluation period, and written testing and written performance evaluations should be performed every 6 months, beginning with the date of the communicator's first regularly scheduled shift worked after her/his release as a primary medical dispatcher. Strict adherence to these quality assurance guidelines will accomplish the function of monitoring the progress of the new communicator, and will ensure that her/his performance continues to meet or exceed accepted standards.

If, during initial training, written examination and/or interim performance evaluation scores fail to meet minimum passing requirements, the recommendation must be made that the trainee repeat all or part of the training process; the evaluation process must also be repeated. If, at the conclusion of the retraining and re-evaluation process, the trainee cannot earn passing scores in all areas of expertise, her/his participation in the communications training program must be terminated.

## WRITTEN MEDICAL COMMUNICATOR EXAMINATIONS: ESTABLISHING A SYSTEM TO EVALUATE TECHNICAL KNOWLEDGE

To realistically measure and evaluate the knowledge base and technical competency level of any communicator, some type of consistent testing must be administered. A comprehensive database must be accumulated containing questions and answers pertaining to all aspects of the medical dispatcher's job duties. This information can be maintained in written form, although it is infinitely easier to store testing material in a simple, user-friendly database program that will run on a personal computer. Regularly scheduled written examinations serve many purposes in the communications center. By accurately analyzing test scores, you can objectively set standards and *prove, in the form of hard-copy documentation, that your dispatchers are qualified to perform their jobs*. You can identify areas where concentration is needed for continuing education. You can compare the performance of one dispatcher with another. You can measure progress, predict future training budget requirements, and significantly increase both the self-confidence and comfort levels of employees in the communications center.

To compile and administer examinations in a rational manner, testing material must be categorized in two ways. First it must be classified by subject. These are some suggested *subject sections* by which to classify your testing material:

**Section 1: Spelling and Dictation.** The most fair and efficient way to administer this section is to prepare a short audio tape on which the speaker says a series of words, phrases, numbers, and common addresses within the service area. Set your own standards for elapsed time between voice signals. The employee listens to the information given and then has a consistent number of seconds to write or type the information correctly. For example, the test administrator gives the participants general instructions for this section of the test, and then plays a prepared audio tape. The voice on the tape says, "1321 North Main." Ten seconds elapse; the voice on the tape says, "Quiet approach requested." Ten seconds elapse, and another voice signal is given. Each employee records the information heard on the tape. Phrases or addresses are given only once. This method measures the employee's ability to hear and understand information, record the information accurately, and spell it correctly.

**Section 2: Mathematics and Calculation.** A series of mathematical problems in varying degrees of difficulty are presented in written form. Problems requiring simple and complex addition, subtraction, multiplication, and division are included. This section measures basic mathematical skills.

**Section 3: Communication.** Subjects evaluated include basic communications theory, basic and advanced telecommunications techniques, telephone techniques, interpersonal relationships, and so on. Varying formats are used, including matching, listing, fill-in-the-blank, and multiple choice. These measure basic and advanced communications skills.

**Section 4: Geographic Knowledge.** Includes, at various levels, response districts or zones, commonly known addresses, landmarks, highways and cross streets, and telephone exchanges in relation to geographic location. Measures ability to pre-alert and dispatch the appropriate unit, provide routing instructions, and so on. Various formats are used.

**Section 5: Medical.** Includes field patient care protocols, medical interrogation protocols, telephone triage, and pre-arrival instruction protocols. Various formats are used, and difficulty increases with the level of the examination. Measures ability to provide "zero minute" response times, respond to patients' medical needs, function within proscribed standards, and participate in field quality assurance programs.

**Section 6: System Status Management.** Includes common terms and definitions, goals, guidelines for unit selection, deployment strategies, documentation techniques, factors impacting system status and system compliance. Measures ability to function within prescribed standards, reduce response delays, maintain system compliance, and understand the consequences of each action taken by the communicator. Various formats are used.

**Section 7: Medicolegal Aspects/Policies and Procedures.** Includes terms and concepts, safeguards, legally appropriate actions, general position statements, specific procedures. Various formats used. Measures retention and decision-making skills and identifies "risk-takers."

**Section 8: Equipment.** Includes types of communications equipment in use in the system, equipment operation, basic troubleshooting techniques, equipment failure notification and repair procedures, and manual "back-up" systems. Various formats used. Measures technical knowledge, decisionmaking, and performance under stress.

Levels of Testing

Testing material must be further classified by *degree of difficulty*. The definition of at least four difficulty levels is recommended; in some extremely complex or "old" systems, more may be required.

*Level 1* tests are entry-level written examinations. Questions are selected from a pool of knowledge easily accessible to any employee of the system. Information is oriented more to the field perspective than specifically to the perspective of the communicator. Emphasis is placed on geographic knowledge of the service area and procedures utilized by medical dispatchers as they directly impact the work performance of field personnel. The basic ability of the candidate to give remote intervention instructions is tested. Questions are formatted as multiple choice, matching, and fill-in-the-blank. Geographic questions are geared to commonly known landmarks and major streets and intersections.

*Level 2* tests are administered at the end of the candidate's initial training period and before her/his final evaluation shifts. Emphasis is slightly shifted to encompass knowledge specifically required of the system status controller. Theoretical information is included, and the SSC's required knowledge of mechanical and technical skills is evaluated. Geographical questions now refer to specific addresses and less commonly recognized landmarks. Formats resemble those found in Level 1 exams, with a slightly higher number of questions that require situational expertise and judgment.

*Level 3* tests are given upon completion of the dispatcher's first 6 months in place following her/his release to work as a primary communicator and assignment to a regularly scheduled shift. Skills levels in advanced intervention and medical interrogation techniques are evaluated. Also included are mechanical knowledge and hardware support. Geographical questions refer to more obscure locations that are usually only learned after both training and time on the job have been completed. More detailed listing, more complex situations, and questions requiring sophisticated, experienced judgment are included.

*Level 4* tests are administered every 6 months to every communicator who has been in place one year or longer. All aspects of the medical communicator's job duties are included. Advanced theoretical knowledge is required. All questioning formats are utilized, with emphasis on complex circumstances, complicated call prioritization and remote intervention instructions, refined judgment skills, and "What if?" situations.

Several different tests for each level can be compiled by extracting different, specially targeted questions from the database. The testing and retesting process serves not only to evaluate the communicator's skills levels and identify the need for additional training or retraining, but also to teach. Study sessions should precede and feedback sessions should follow the administration of each exam.

Again, possible earned points from each test should equal a minimum of 500. "Bonus" questions, either unrelated to medical communications or inappropriately advanced for the level of exam being administered, may be included on each test. Available points from extra credit questions should not exceed 10.

If the desire is to test a greater body of knowledge in a particular area, more emphasis can be placed on one subject category by *increasing the number of questions* in a section while *decreasing their point value* (see Figure 16.5). For example, 35 questions about geographic knowledge worth 5 points each yield a total of 175 points for the section, and account for 35 percent of the total available points for the exam. If you want to ask more questions in this subject category, you may *increase* the number of questions to 175, while *decreasing* the value of each to 1 point. Total points possible in this section remain at 175, which continues to conform to the suggested 35 percent subject distribution.

| Subject Section | Level of Difficulty (%) | | | |
|---|---|---|---|---|
| | 1 | 2 | 3 | 4 |
| 1. Spelling/dictation | 15 | 10 | 10 | 10 |
| 2. Math/calculation | 15 | 10 | 10 | 10 |
| 3. Communication | 5 | 10 | 10 | 10 |
| 4. Geographic | 35 | 25 | 20 | 20 |
| 5. Medical | 15 | 15 | 20 | 20 |
| 6. System status management | 5 | 10 | 10 | 10 |
| 7. Medicolegal aspects policies and procedures | 5 | 10 | 10 | 10 |
| 8. Equipment | 5 | 10 | 10 | 10 |
| | 100 | 100 | 100 | 100 |

Figure 16.5 *Suggested distribution of examination questions by subject category and level of difficulty. Each level of examination includes no fewer than 500 available points. A high standard of deviation in distribution is seen in Level 1 testing; distribution is gradually equalized as testing progresses through Level 4. Final emphasis remains on medical expertise and geograpic knowledge of the service area.*

## OTHER TYPES OF TESTING

### Psychological Testing

Attempts to document reliable methods for applying broad psychological principles to the general public began when the first formal psychological research laboratory was established by Wilhelm Wundt in 1879. Studies show that psychological testing is primarily useful in isolating and identifying *undesirable* traits in the individuals evaluated, rather than in recognizing general positive principles. As soon as a study is published establishing what is presented as a "solid" theory of behavior patterns or characteristics with measurable results, another set of statistics proves it incorrect. Even when testing is conducted by professional agencies trained to evaluate psychological traits and aptitudes in the business setting, the results are open to a large degree of interpretation. Professional psychologists have been struggling with the process for more than a hundred years now, and they haven't completely figured it out yet. I wouldn't hold my breath, and I would *never* exclusively rely on the results of testing of this type.

### Intelligence Testing

Tests designed to measure and score intelligence are also largely open to interpretation, and therefore to misinterpretation. The general public routinely misunderstands the results of these tests. Most people also attach far too much importance to them. If I could "prove" to you with a set of numbers that you were stupid, would you still be able to find your way to work each morning? Outside a research facility, in the real world, test results must be *objective and clearly measurable*; they must show a *relationship* to have any practical meaning.

## ATTITUDE SURVEYS

One type of written feedback that *is* useful in our industry is the general attitude survey. These can, and should, be completed regularly by applicants to the communications training program, medical dispatchers, field personnel, and managers. The results of these polls can identify training needs, indicate the status of confidence and morale, and lead managers to isolate and correct problems *before* they reach a critical level.

One important note: if your desire is to obtain an *accurate* picture of how your co-workers feel about your system, *the timing of the survey is very important*. While it is usually most convenient for managers or supervisors to have employees complete the survey information at the same time their performance appraisals are performed, this usually won't reflect a true picture of the employees' attitudes. When completing a survey just prior to a performance evaluation, the employee may unconsciously project a more positive attitude than she or he really feels. When the survey is completed immediately following an evaluation, the employee may project a more negative outlook than she or he usually feels (out of anger or resentment felt over an unsatisfactory performance evaluation), or a more positive attitude than is realistically felt (out of "gratitude" or a feeling of obligation following the completion of a satisfactory evaluation).

## ANALYZING AND INTERPRETING TEST RESULTS: ESTABLISHING THE PROPER PERSPECTIVE

The ways in which examination scores are evaluated and used are probably more important than the test questions themselves. If the results are not properly utilized, the figures are arbitrary and meaningless. The most practical use of test scores lies in establishing relationships.

### Measures of Relationship: Common Terms

These words and definitions are commonly used in analyzing test scores and evaluating their meanings.

**Validation.** When the average instructor, student, trainee or employee thinks of "validating a test," she/he thinks in terms of whether a particular question is "good" or "bad." *Validation* is actually the process of deciding whether or not the question really measures what it was intended to measure (see Figure 16.6). Does a question

**Medical Communicator General Knowledge Exam 1.02**
*March 27*

| Employee | Test Score |
|----------|-----------|
| 1 | 88 |
| 2 | 63 |
| 3 | 77 |
| 4 | 88 |
| 5 | 95 |
| 6 | 91 |
| 7 | 91 |
| 8 | 92 |
| 9 | 64 |
| 10 | 91 |
| Total | 840 |

Figure 16.6 *In this display of test scores, 10 employees were given identical examinations. 840 (the sum of all the test scores added together) divided by 10 (the number of participants in the testing) = 84. This is the mean. The two middle scores are 88 and 91; the middle point between these two scores = 89.5. This is the median. The test score earned by the most people (the most common score) = 91. This is the mode.*

measure the participant's knowledge of a subject, *or the participant's ability to comprehend an overly complicated testing format*? If 95 percent of those taking a particular test mark a question incorrectly, does this mean that the question was poorly phrased, or that a general area of knowledge is critically deficient?

In our profession, the acceptable margin for error is very small; our patients' lives depend on our ability to consistently provide excellent performance. Generally, using our frame of reference and understanding the rigid standards for our performance, negative test results are not sufficient reason to "throw out" or disqualify a series of questions or a subject category of knowledge.

**Mean.** The *mean* is what most of us call the *average* of a set of numbers. Mathematicians and statisticians know this number as the *arithmetic mean*. The mean is calculated by adding all the test scores together and dividing that total by the number of persons taking the test (see Figure 16.7).

**Median.** The *median* (Figure 16.7) is simply the *middle* score in any distribution, or the point between the two middle scores. The median can indicate much more than just the result of a mathematical computation. It can help you to discover and identify a general attitude, perception, misperception, social standard, or locally held view. While the median is frequently not of great use statistically, it can, in combination with the *mode*, identify the social attitude that occupies the "middle of the road."

**Standard Deviation of Test Scores**
**Medical Communicator General Knowledge Exam 1.03**
**March 27**

| Employee | Test Score | Deviation From Mean | Squared Deviation |
|---|---|---|---|
| 1 | 88 | +4 | 16 |
| 2 | 63 | -21 | 441 |
| 3 | 77 | -7 | 49 |
| 4 | 88 | +4 | 16 |
| 5 | 95 | +11 | 121 |
| 6 | 91 | +7 | 49 |
| 7 | 91 | +7 | 49 |
| 8 | 92 | +8 | 64 |
| 9 | 64 | -20 | 400 |
| 10 | 91 | +7 | 49 |
| | 840 | | 1254 |

Figure 16.7 *The* mean *is 840 divided by 10 = 84. Subtract 84 from each test score. This is the* deviation. *Square the absolute value (no - or +). This is the* squared deviation. *Now divide the total from the squared deviation column by the number of participants. 1254 divided by 10 = 125.4. This is the* variance. The standard deviation is the square root of the variance. Standard deviation for this group of test scores is 11.2

**Mode.** The *mode* is another very useful social indicator (Figure 16.7). It is simply the *most common* score, or the score made by the greatest number of persons. In any set of test results where no two scores are identical, the mode will be absent.

**Central Tendency.** The *central tendency* is sometimes very clear, and sometimes ambiguous and hard to define. It implies the *general inclination* of the group being tested. Arriving at the identification of a central tendency may incorporate the use of the mean, the median, the mode, or all three, depending on the area of general knowledge being tested, the test being given, and how the numbers will be used. In any distribution that is completely "normal" by statistical definition, the mean, median, and mode will be the same.

Measures of Variability

**The Range.** How much of a point spread is there in the distribution of a set of test scores? The mathematical difference between the highest and lowest scores is the *range*. This figure is frequently misused, since it can allow a single high or low score to carry too much weight. For example, let's say 10 dispatchers are each given an identical examination. If the two highest grades are 98 and 88, and the two lowest scores are 72 and 50, would the range be an accurate indicator of how much these dispatchers know? By definition, the range in this case is the difference between 98 and 50, or 48 points. However, the *next* highest and lowest scores are 88 and 72, which gives a difference of only 16 points. Since the remaining six scores are clustered between 87 and 71, the range is not a true indicator of the communicators' knowledge. It is misleading. A better method to gauge variability is to calculate the *standard deviation*.

Standard Deviation from Mean

This is a practical way to view test results, since it measures the amount of positive and negative deviation from the *mean*, or average (Figure 16.7).

Each score in the distribution contributes to the standard deviation. Therefore, extremely low or high scores do not inappropriately impact the final figure. Standard deviation may be large or small, depending on how closely the scores cluster around the mean.

## TRAINING, RETRAINING, AND CONTINUING EDUCATION

While initial training, remedial retraining of in-place communicators, and continuing education for medical dispatchers all involve the acquisition of knowledge, the specific needs for each category are unique. Each must approached in a slightly different manner.

### Initial Training

Careful planning must be completed before the actual training process ever begins. You must identify knowledge categories and acceptable competency levels for communicators in your system. Accurate, thorough documentation must be provided of the time spent training for each job task. The degree of competency observed should be noted at intervals lasting a maximum of 2 weeks throughout the length of the employee's initial training. At the end of the initial training period, the trainee should be evaluated by the department manager or administrator. I suggest that trainees be required to perform all job tasks correctly 90–95 percent of the time before they are released to work unsupervised and in a primary position. In-place communicators should also be required to consistently perform at this 90–95 percent accuracy level. *This is a tough standard to meet; however, there's not a lot of room for mistakes in a medical dispatch center.* Requiring an accuracy level of 90 percent or better will also improve your system's position if a communicator should be accused of improper actions or named as the defendant in civil litigation. This departmental requirement demonstrates a high level of effort on the part of the system or service to ensure the delivery of the best possible patient care.

Teaching techniques used with the new trainee must be basic and simple; a step-by-step process should be followed. Simple tasks are learned first, progressing with time to more difficult responsibilities. A typical advancement program might begin with relaying medical information and progress through nonemergency call-taking, emergency call-taking, and finally radio operation and management of system status. Ideally, the communicator acting as trainer should have no other tasks than to teach.

The trainee should first observe a primary communicator performing a function. This observation can only be effective if the trainee hears everything the primary dispatcher hears. *Teaching headsets or mutually accessible telephones are suggested.* The primary dispatcher should explain each procedure immediately after it is performed. The trainee may then perform the task, supervised by the communicator acting as trainer. *Again, trainer supervision can only be accomplished if the trainer hears everything the trainee hears.* Teaching headsets, dual console headset jacks, or mutually accessible telephones are required. When the trainer is supervising the trainee's performance as radio operator, an audible external speaker may be used. Finally, the trainer should "sign off" on the procedure; when this occurs, the trainer signifies (and is willing to put it in writing) that the trainee is qualified to perform the task without the direct supervision previously required at the console.

### Remedial Retraining

When, through testing and interim performance evaluations, a deficit or "weak point" is identified in a medical dispatcher's performance, the obvious need is for that performance to improve.

Historically, we have identified the problem area, instructed the communicator to resolve the problem or improve the performance, and then been surprised when no improvement occurred. In some systems, disciplinary action is the first remedial step taken by managers or supervisors. Ideally, the communicator should be trained, not punished; for obvious, lasting refinement of communications skills to take place, the dispatcher must be provided with suggestions for how to improve, and with examples of successful job performance.

## Continuing Education

The completion of a designated number of recertification and/or continuing education hours is routinely required for continued certification of EMS personnel. With organization and pre-approval from your system's clinical and training coordinators and your state health department or board, your medical dispatchers can complete their CE hour requirements for maintaining certification while simultaneously ensuring that their performance in the communications center remains sharp.

**Providing the Information.** Special "schools" or training sessions don't have to be developed by supervisors or managers; they don't have to cost a ton of money. The most effective sessions with the greatest amount of usable, practical information are frequently coordinated and presented by the line communicators themselves.

Many benefits follow when line employees actively participate in improving the knowledge base of the entire communications department. When you research your subject, plan and schedule your own presentation, and actually deliver the material, you learn much more than if the information is simply handed to you. You learn research techniques and time and organizational structure; you improve your public speaking skills and poise. Your confidence level increases as your knowledge grows.

How do you start? *First, identify a need.* From test results or interviewing your co-workers, identify a subject category where the comfort level is low, or where general knowledge could be improved. (Note that your subject should be of general interest or address a departmental need, rather than just reflect one of your "pet peeves.") Then just dig in and research the subject. It may be that the dispatchers in your system routinely operate "blind" when assigning units to calls in a certain remote part of your service area. Because the call volume is low in that sector, the opportunity has not arisen during normal work hours for the communicators to become thoroughly familiar with the geography of the area. You can contact the county or parish surveyor's office for that area and request current maps. You can redraw maps with major structures and routing hazards identified. You can speak with city officials in the area, and build street guides from the information they can provide. You can print up your own list of major intersections and dispatching considerations.

When you know everything there is to know about your subject, it's time to organize your presentation. You should provide training information both in the form of an oral or verbal presentation, and with printed material.

The oral or verbal presentation should be the *primary* source of information. It offers a face-to-face forum, and gives both the instructor and the students *the opportunities to speak and to listen*. These are some points to consider when preparing for an oral presentation:

- *The key word is prepare. Organize your material.* Decide which information is really important, and which is more than your co-workers need to know. (Even I believe that it's theoretically possible to have too much information.) Write down in outline form what you want to relate. Make the progression logical and orderly, allowing for a smooth, continuous flow.
- *Structure the time carefully.* State clearly the time when the class or study session will begin, and when it will end. Don't start late, and don't let the session drag on forever. If you've organized carefully enough, you will be able to start and end the session on time.
- *Retain control of what the time is used for.* Don't allow the training class to turn into a general forum for complaints. If the need is identified for a general "bitch" session, then ask that the department manager schedule time specifically for that purpose. If, because of a very recent, very unusual event, there is the need for some immediate venting by the group, make sure it takes place *before* the training session begins.
- *Don't just read* your notes or the printed material you have compiled to be distributed. Medical communicators are adults; if they want to read the printed material, they can do that for themselves.
- *Make sure that the training session takes place in a comfortable setting* (plenty of room, not too hot or too cold, etc.). Arrange things so that your group won't be disturbed (unless, of course, a major incident takes place in your service area during class time — and if you *are* disturbed, it had better be *really* major).
- *Move around while you talk.* Use visual aids: an overhead projector, large, easy-to-read charts, a blackboard. Intelligent people frequently get bored easily. You have to do something to hold the group's attention. If you don't provide enough diversion to keep things interesting, the lunatics will take over the asylum.
- *Keep the presentation short.* More than 2 hours is too long. One-hour sessions are better.
- *Allow time for breaks* if the presentation runs an hour or longer.
- *Allow access by all communications personnel.* If your system has lots of money, you can videotape the session and play it for those who were working when the presentation was made. Otherwise,

plan for two sessions, one at the beginning of the week and one at the end; all communicators should have the opportunity to attend.

The other critical component in the information presentation process is the provision of printed material. Just telling people about something isn't enough; if you want the information to be recalled and used consistently, the communicators should be given handouts to take away with them. When organizing handout material, you should consider these things:

- *Again, organize.* Provide a cover sheet stating what the handout is, and what's included in it.
- *If the material to be presented is complex, divide it into sections or subheadings by subject.*
- *Highlight important words*, phrases, concepts, lists of items. If you are typing the handouts on a typewriter, personal computer, or word processor, you can accomplish this with bold or italic print or inset margins, for example.
- *Include charts*, graphs, maps, illustrations, and examples, especially when numbers are involved. (How many times have you understood a concept or a procedure perfectly in class, only to get home and find it made no sense at all?)
- *Print your material in a simple, easy-to-read typeface* with sufficient space in the margins and between the lines to make notes.
- *Don't print everything!* This printed material is meant to be a *supplemental* learning tool; the primary source of knowledge is you and the personal instruction you can provide.
- *Number the pages.* Make sure the pages are correctly collated, and that there is a copy for everyone.

The trick to making a program like this work is to devise a schedule, and then stick to it. If you are the department manager, take into consideration suggestions by the communicators themselves; then identify a planned number of training hours to be available each month (1 hour, 2 hours, 4 hours). Set regularly scheduled days for training (for example, the first Tuesday and Thursday of every month). Outline subject categories that need to be covered. Then let each dispatcher choose a subject and a month in which to present an informational review and update. Using this type of plan, training schedules can easily be set for up to a year at a time.

## AUDIO TAPE REVIEWS

Another regularly scheduled type of training and feedback can be accomplished by establishing an audio tape review committee. One of the best training tools available to the medical communicator is the audio tape of that employee performing her or his job duties. Many, many times, we have no idea how we actually sound to other people.

Medical communicators can be appointed on a rotating basis to a continually functioning tape review committee. Any dispatcher in good standing in the department should be eligible and all should be required to participate in the program. Since alternates (part-time communicators) are required to have both an understanding of system operation and competency levels equal to those of full-time dispatchers, alternates should also be required to participate in the process; however, demands on alternates' time must be structured to be less than that on full-time dispatchers. If, due to call volume and the work load in the communications center, the time required to perform tape reviews is not available during regularly scheduled shifts, the SSCs may complete the process during their primary call-back shifts. (While the primary call-back or standby procedure is frequently used in the field setting, this is another principle routinely omitted in planning communications center operations. Establishing an on-call process for the dispatch center can dramatically reduce scrambling to staff shifts left open by absences with last-minute notifications.)

A specific number of full-time and alternate dispatchers may be scheduled to serve on the tape review committee each calendar month. When structured on a monthly schedule, their period of service can begin on the first day of the month and end with the last. One communicator or a team of communicators, whether full-time or an alternate, may be designated to be audited each calendar week. During that week, the communicators being audited keep a log sheet documenting the date and times spent in each working position in the communications center. The following week, the tape review committee listens to master tapes for the appropriate time period and, via the reel-to-reel playback equipment, locates voice recordings of the designated communicator:

- Receiving and processing information for ten nonemergency calls
- Receiving and processing information for ten emergency calls, including prioritization questions and answers and remote intervention instructions
- Acting as radio operator for a period of not less than 2 hours

These voice transmissions can be rerecorded onto a cassette tape and marked for identification with the name of the dispatcher being evaluated, the dates and times of the events, the incident numbers, and the names of the tape review committee members involved.

When the required voice transmissions have been recorded onto cassette, the committee members, together or separately as schedules permit, complete written tape review reports for calls received or dispatched by the communicator whose job performance is being reviewed. Each time there is a behavioral deviation from in-place protocols, the committee should send an interdepartmental request for additional information to the clinical division (see Figure 16.8). The clinical coordinator should return the report with written documentation of the actual situation that existed on the scene, as reported by the field care-givers. This report will enable the committee to compare

| REQUEST FOR CLINICAL INFORMATION ||
|---|---|
| From: Communications Division | To: Clinical Division |
| Request Routed To: | Date Sent: |
| Person Requesting Information (Return To): ||
| Incident #:    Incident Date: | Unit(s): |
| Encounter Address: ||
| Call-Taker(s): | Dispatcher: |
| Field Response Team(s): ||
| Problem Encountered: ||
| Information Requested: ||
| Received in Clinical Division By: | Date: |
| Clinical Division Reply: ||
| Returned to Communications By: | Date: |
| Routed To:    Received In Communications By: ||
| Date Reply Received: | Reviewed By: |

Figure 16.8  *Request for clinical information*

what was said to the call-taker with how the call was prioritized and dispatched, and to compare both of these with the real situation found. With this procedure in place, medical dispatchers quickly get a *realistic* picture of their own call-taking, interviewing, and prioritization skills.

Group participation is an invaluable tool with which to facilitate quality assurance. In each evaluation, both the dispatcher being audited and the committee members performing the review will learn and improve their skills. Group involvement also helps to establish or reaffirm the existence of and compliance with reasonable performance standards for the department. However, when the process logically progresses to the point where remedial training and/or disciplinary action is indicated, the "buck" has to stop with one person. Therefore, the final evaluation of information provided by the tape review committee, along with any remedial retraining or disciplinary action, must be the sole responsibility of the communications department manager. Although the knowledge and insights gained in the audit process may be shared among the controllers, remedial or disciplinary action taken by the communications manager or supervisor must, as always, remain confidential.

## ROUTINE PERFORMANCE EVALUATIONS

Comprehensive written performance evaluations must be conducted with each fully trained, regularly assigned full-time and alternate medical communicator; these evaluations should be performed by the communications director or manager at intervals not to exceed 6 months. Attendance and tardiness records, typing test results, written communications examination scores, written interim evaluations, the results of audio tape reviews, response time compliance percentages, and generally observed attitudes, motivation, and cooperation skills should all be considered. The evaluation process must include discussion time with the dispatcher and an opportunity for the employee to document in writing her or his response to the findings of the evaluation. Each completed evaluation form, along with recommendations for rate increases as applicable, should be forwarded to the chief or chief executive officer for review. Any communicator who disagrees with the content of a performance evaluation, or otherwise disagrees with any attitude or action of the department manager, must be allowed to directly contact the chief or CEO, without fear of retaliation, for discussion and resolution of the problem.

## SUMMARY AND REVIEW

1. Why is there a need for quality assurance in the medical dispatch center?

2. What factors have caused the need for quality control in emergency medical service to increase over the last few years?

3. How is the team approach useful in providing quality assurance?

4. What are the two types of errors committed in the medical communications center?

5. Define medical control.

6. What are the benefits of standardizing your telephone procedures? Does your system utilize procedural standardization? What are the obvious dangers when protocols are not established and standardized?

7. What is the difference between a general position statement and a specific policy or procedure?

8. How, when, and why are new employees identified and selected to work in your dispatch center? Are the practices in place in your system sound or unsound?

9. What kind of testing is required as part of your division's hiring process?

10. How are strengths, weaknesses, and general progress documented for trainees in your communications department?

11. Define the following statistical terms:

| | |
|---|---|
| Validation | Mean |
| Median | Mode |
| Central tendency | Range |
| Standard deviation from mean | |

12. What are the three categories of concern in the educational process for medical communicators?

# Chapter 17

# STRESS MANAGEMENT FOR THE MEDICAL COMMUNICATOR

*"One day soon, I shall burst this bud
of calm and blossom into hysteria."*
— *Unknown*

COMPONENTS OF THE STRESS REACTION

The position of medical communicator is one of the most critically important positions in our entire industry. As a professional medical dispatcher, you are literally responsible for managing every detail of the working status of an entire emergency medical response system. The burden of responsibility involved in successfully performing this function is great; the accompanying stress can be overwhelming.

While a certain amount of stress is inherent in any profession, medical communicators seem to overload more quickly than employees in other types of business; therefore, it's important that we become proficient at identifying and managing unsatisfactorily high stress levels and burnout. There are three major components to any good, workable stress management program. The first is an understanding of what "stress" is. What causes it? Are there good and bad kinds of stress? How can we avoid stress?

The second component involves recognizing the signs of actual or impending stress overload and identifying unacceptable stress levels. Before we can find a solution to a problem, we must recognize that the problem exists. What factors are routinely identified as impacting the stress levels of medical dispatchers? What are the danger signs that a controller's stress level is becoming too high?

The final component of a successful stress management system is the identification and explanation of available mechanisms to deal with stress, both in and away from the communications center. In any system, there are always a number of options available, ranging from simple personal techniques to professional counseling.

## WHAT IS STRESS?

Simply stated, *stress is the body's reaction to a basic need*. It is a safety mechanism. For example, if the temperature is too cold, the body tells us to seek warmth. Thus, we prevent permanent tissue damage or death from cold exposure. If a noise is too loud, we move away from it or cover our ears. We avoid damage to our hearing. We react automatically to constant changes in our environment, and "environment" can include merely physical considerations, or may also include our mental status, our emotional state, or the social situation in which we find ourselves. Stress can be physical, mental, emotional, social, or environmental. Any factor that causes a stress-type reaction is called a *stressor*.

A certain amount of stress is normal in our day-to-day lives. It is a warning sign; it keeps us from hurting ourselves. When stress becomes unmanageable or impairs work performance, we can modify our behavior and responses and/or make changes in our physical and social environments to avoid or decrease *stress overload*. If stress overload is not identified and managed successfully, *burnout* will inevitably follow.

Burnout occurs in stages. It is usually difficult to define, even harder to recognize, and, for the vast majority of us who have not received specific training in the area, impossible to successfully manage alone. Burnout in the area of medical communications is as hard to define as it is in any other industry. To further complicate the problem, professional medical dispatchers seem to be at a higher risk for burnout than employees in most other vocations. The best and most successful medical dispatchers put their hearts and souls into their work. When you make this kind of emotional and intellectual investment day after day and do not learn to manage the stressors inherent in your work, *you will eventually emotionally burn out. It's a matter of time.*

It is important to understand that each person is an individual, and each reacts to stress differently. The stressors that overload one person may actually be enjoyable for another. It is virtually impossible to set rigid rules to deal with different types of stress.

## REINFORCING OUR PUBLIC IMAGE

We in emergency medical service believe that we have an image to maintain. We are the people who can handle anything. We can hold ourselves together and continue to function when everyone around us is falling apart. We can look at blood and broken human bodies day after day without it dragging us down. We shut ourselves off from the sadness inherent in our jobs, and compensate with all-too-familiar "gallows humor." This notion of invincibility is reinforced every time a friend, acquaintance, or family member says to us, "I could never do what you do for a living." The more we're told that we are special, the more pressure we feel to avoid any display that might be interpreted as weakness.

Well, get a clue, okay? Sooner or later, you'll have to consciously realize that you deal with pain, loss, grief, death and dying every single day that you work. *Nobody* can do that without it having some effect on them. At some point, we have to leave behind this "macho" image we've created for ourselves. It must be well understood that there should never be any embarrassment associated with acknowledging that your individual stress level is unacceptably high, or in seeking assistance to help you deal with your stress. EMS professionals are strong and resourceful and capable; they are also *human*.

## COMMON STRESS FACTORS FOR MEDICAL COMMUNICATORS

You love your job, right? This position challenges you in ways you've never been challenged before; at the end of your shift, you usually go home feeling like you've really accomplished something. You love your family, your friends, your hobbies, and your home. The feelings of responsibility and authority that you've learned to welcome in the course of doing your job have spilled over into your activities away from work; others see you as successful and in charge of your life. So why do you feel the way you do so often?

Why do tears come to your eyes so easily? Why do you feel so often that you've somehow let down or short-changed both your family and your co-workers? Why can't you get out of bed in the morning? Why are you always so tired? Why don't you want to come to work? While there is always the possibility that you have contracted some rare tropical disease (and everyone will be sorry when they find out you're really ill), the answer is probably as simple as *stress overload and burnout*.

Health care providers in all fields and at all levels now accept as fact the impact that mental and emotional stress have on the occurrence and progression of physical disease. The evidence also indicates that we can learn to successfully and effectively manage stress overload and avoid burnout altogether. With training, we can learn to keep our stress levels within an acceptable range. The first step to positive stress management is the identification of stressors already recognized as impacting others in your chosen field. These are some of the stress factors that will eventually affect you as you work as a medical communicator:

**The Hours You Work.** By its very nature, our business operates 24 hours a day, 7 days a week, 52 weeks a year. This sets the medical communicator apart from the general public, which works largely a "normal" work week, 0900 to 1700, Monday through Friday. Our schedules make arranging other, unrelated social activities difficult; conflicts between our scheduled shifts and the time demands of family and school may appear irreconcilable.

**The Inconsistency of Demands for Action.** At certain times in the communications center, there seems to be more work to be done than can possibly be accomplished by the medical dispatchers on duty. At other times, the activity level drops to almost zero. Having been cautioned about the dangers of allowing your concentration level to slip, you attempt to maintain an energy level sufficient to deal effectively with any new occurrence. This sporadic type of stimulation feels like an emotional roller coaster ride. *(Get ready . . . Do something! Never mind . . . Get ready . . . Do something! Never mind . . . .)* Until any communicator's behavioral patterns are adjusted to compensate for this fluctuation in demand, the marked differences between overload and underload will cause mental and emotional stress which may be translated into fatigue and actual physical illness.

When the pace in the dispatch center picks up, you are required to perform many tasks at once. This, like many other identifiable prerequisites for medical dispatching, is a natural talent; it cannot be taught. While the possession of this ability is a natural source of pride for the medical dispatcher, it may cloud your judgment. In times of extreme overload, there may actually *be* more work than you can accomplish effectively. When this happens, most professional communicators will feel dissatisfied with their performance, and their stress levels will go up.

**The Levels of Concentration and Effort.** This is a very intense, demanding job. It requires that you always stay on top of things, and that you never relax. Anything less than 100 percent on your part is unacceptable; lives depend on your level of effort. The hours are usually long, and the performance demands placed on you are rigid and exhausting. Even when you're bone tired, you must achieve absolute, total concentration. I can tell you simultaneously that you *must* give 100 percent all the time, and that *no one* can give 100 percent all the time. *(There now; don't you feel better?)*

Although some field employees may share the same *type* of shifts that we work, we are even more restricted than they in that we must remain alert to deal with the isolated events that take place even when the overall system activity level is slow. We are the stimulant that wakes up the sleeping field crews; we have to be awake and functional *before* they do.

**Emotional Fallout from Co-Workers.** While the scope of total available EMS resources in any service area can be quite vast, as medical communicators we deal primarily with other employees of our own systems: our shift partners, field crew members, and field supervisors. Less frequently we interact with members of first responder agencies and employees of hospitals and treatment facilities. The attitudes and appropriateness of response of these team members profoundly affect our own attitudes and stress levels. When another member of the team displays an unpleasant, unprofessional, or ineffective attitude or response, we are programmed to automatically "kneejerk" and react to that display. If you are continually exposed to partners or field crews who cling to negative attitudes, eventually you will become dissatisfied as well. It's important to remember that the people behind these "voices of doom" may not believe themselves that things are as bad as they make them sound; it could be they just want to bitch.

Many times, the cause of the other team member's attitude is purely personal, and has no relationship with the medical dispatcher at all. If you can remember this, you can condition yourself to minimize your response.

**The Constant Noise.** Almost every piece of equipment in the typical communications center beeps, rings, jingles, or buzzes. These sounds are important signals to alert us that an event is taking place which requires corresponding action on our part. In addition to their own equipment, dispatchers in many systems are required to monitor radio frequencies in use by other systems or agencies. Some dispatch centers are still positioned in openly accessible areas, and are not even acoustically isolated. The communicators who work in these facilities catch the audio clutter and "fallout" from surrounding areas.

When several telephone lines ring at once, bells and buzzers are going off, crews on the primary dispatch channel are attempting to contact the radio operator, the medic waiting on a specialty channel is screaming for attention, and personnel from another agency are handling a multiple-alarm fire response on an additional radio frequency, it is a natural reaction to become "rattled." I believe the ability to deal effectively with a large number of different audio stimulation sources at once is another example of an inborn talent; you either have it or you don't. Many people can never master this task.

**Environmental Control.** In some communications centers, the mechanisms that control noise, temperature and lighting levels of the dispatchers' work area are located outside the work area itself. Although this may at first seem to be a minor source of irritation, physical discomfort can accumulate and combine with other stressors to create an overall stress level that is intolerably high.

**Confinement in the Work Area.** When working in the field, there is a great deal of freedom of movement. Even when assigned to a small, restricted posting area, the crew still has the choice to remain still, to drive around, to stay in the unit, to go into a fire station or place of business, and so on. In the dispatch center, we are tied by our headset connecting cords to our consoles, or to a telephone system for the majority of our shifts. This lack of freedom of movement can, as previously discussed, combine with other physical and mental stressors to increase overall stress to unacceptable levels.

**Media Attention and High Visibility to the Public.** Even

when the communicator knows that a call is routine, if a media representative calls and requests information about that call, it appears in a different light. The knowledge that media agencies are scanning your radio channels adds a certain importance to the event. Any good radio operator can, with practice, delude herself or himself into believing that only the system's field crews are listening to the radio transmissions. When the fact that other agencies are listening is brought home, the actions of the dispatcher seem to take on added importance. Just knowing that "outsiders" are listening can make you nervous. Once again, stress levels increase.

**Intense Emotional Involvement.** This stressor has only been identified relatively recently, as more and more systems become involved in medical prioritization and giving pre-arrival instructions. The medical dispatcher bonds, quickly and out of necessity, with the caller in crisis. Many times this personal investment on the part of the controller is the *only* factor that allows her or him to break through the caller's hysteria and provide life-saving intervention. When a call in which the dispatcher has invested emotionally has a happy ending, the feedback is positive. You come away from the experience feeling good, proud of yourself and of the job that you do. When the end result of a call is negative, the residual feeling that stays with the communicator is correspondingly negative. In those infrequent cases where, no matter how diligent the effort, the call-taker simply cannot influence the caller enough to control and direct the situation, a feeling of failure results. In addition, there will always be particular types of incidents, voice characteristics, accents, words, or phrases that will trigger an unpleasant personal memory for a particular communicator, and thus key an angry, frustrated, or unhappy emotional response. Because we cannot call "time out" to deal with the emotions of the moment, they frequently become buried; because they have not been successfully dealt with, they become part of the emotional baggage that contributes to and exacerbates stress reactions.

**A Lack of Options.** Many of the personnel who are employed in the emergency medical dispatch center began their careers on the field side of the business. Some moved into communications because of physical injuries which prevented them from continuing in an operations capacity; others became bored or burned out with field work. Whatever the reason for the move, many of these professionals now feel that they do not have the option to return to the field setting. For ex-field and for other types of communications personnel, stressors common to other industries, such as the fear and disruption involved in finding another job, come into play. If you seek other employment because you're unhappy in your communications job, will you have to change your schedule? You will certainly lose all your seniority; will you have to take a cut in pay? Will you have to interview or take a test? What if you fail?

It has been my experience that people become their most miserable, and frequently their most irrational, when they feel they are out of options. As a very smart old man once told me, "You can back a coward into a corner, but you don't have to like it."

## SIGNS AND SYMPTOMS OF STRESS OVERLOAD AND BURNOUT

*Stress overload and burnout are processes, not events.* They happen gradually, and build slowly to an unsatisfactory climax. A professional communicator will not, realistically, be "fine" one shift and "crack up" the next. If a dispatcher is out of control today and seemed fine yesterday, it is because no one, including the employee herself/himself, noticed the gradual changes taking place. There are degrees of overload and burnout, and each degree presents with any of a number of identifiers. Individuals may experience slight variations of signs and symptoms described here; the important thing is to watch for and recognize signs and symptoms when they occur, and to stop their progression. To enable you to recognize and treat stress overload *early*, these are some of the questions you should ask yourself and your shift partners:

**Are You Easily Fatigued?** The inability to get over the feeling that you are "always tired" can be a symptom in more than one way. What we interpret as physical fatigue may actually be emotional or mental fatigue translated to the physical by the mind and body. Emotional stress and strain are often felt as physical tiredness. Also, when we are overloaded with mental and/or emotional stress, sleep patterns are easily disturbed. You may be constantly tired because you are genuinely not getting enough sleep.

When you are constantly experiencing feelings of fatigue, you are able to accomplish only the most basic essentials of the communicator's job. The emotional investment that marks the difference between satisfactory and unsatisfactory performance levels is simply an impossibility when you're always exhausted. Support for your co-workers also seems to be more than you can consistently contribute.

**Are You Bored with Your Job?** Human emotions cycle; it's the nature of the animal. Temporary feelings of disillusionment with your job as a reaction to a specific event are normal. Those negative feelings that do not subside after the particular source of irritation is resolved are hallmark signs of stress overload. A transient loss of motivation due to boredom is also normal. However, this is a competitive and rewarding job, if you're suited for it; if you cannot regain your desire to excel, you could be in trouble.

Idealistic, romantic (and sometimes unrealistic) people are more susceptible to burnout than any others. They bring an enormous amount of personal investment to their jobs. They tend to believe that happy endings are directly related to the amount and level of effort they invest in the project. When endings turn out to be unhappy, they, on some level, whether conscious and verbalized or not, assume blame for the outcome. "If I had tried harder, things would have turned out differently"; "If I had thought to say (fill in the blank), maybe she could have followed my pre-arrival instructions." I have observed that the type of personality that tends to assume responsibility for *everything*, whether or not there is actually any direct responsibility for the event (called, in some literature, the "co-dependent personality"), is uniquely drawn to EMS as a profession, and emergency medical dispatching in particular. In order to do this job well and not allow yourself to be "eaten alive" by inappropriate feelings of guilt and failure, you must learn to balance your sense of responsibility between two extremes (not caring at all and caring too much). You are a medical professional and an emergency medical communicator; you are not the master of the universe. You simply cannot hold yourself personally responsible for the state of the entire planet. You *can* study hard, practice, keep your skills levels high, invest enough emotional involvement in your job to perform at 100 percent the majority of the time, and leave the work place at the end of each shift knowing that you have performed a critically important, life-saving and life-changing function, and performed it well.

When the energy level of a beginning controller is very high, expectations are usually also high. (While this phenomenon is most frequently seen in entry-level communicators, it also routinely occurs with those dispatchers who, as a result of intervention by or counseling with an evaluator, have reassessed their performance, and are newly motivated to improve.) With high expectations for our own performance levels comes the expectation of happy endings. When these universally positive outcomes do not come about, the communicator's basic motivation to excel can be lost. Medical dispatchers must learn to pace themselves, and not allow all their emotional resources to be exhausted at once.

### Do You Frequently Experience Negative Feelings About Yourself, Your Job, or Your Employer?

*"Nothing to do but work, nothing to eat but food,
nothing to wear but clothes to keep one from going nude."*
— Ben F. King, "The Pessimist"

A consistently negative attitude is another cardinal sign of potentially critical stress buildup. Changes in attitude usually occur slowly and gradually. Some sources will tell you that this is not an easy sign to recognize. I believe that it's relatively easy to identify those who suffer from persistently negative attitudes: they are those people who constantly whine and complain; they make you lose your mind, and make you want to kill them. When burnout threatens, those who are generally and usually negative in their attitudes will become more so; in this situation, you truly may not notice for quite some time. Those who are usually positive are much more visible in the display of this change. They may make negative remarks that are very uncharacteristic for them. A dispatcher with a negative, bad-tempered attitude not only affects her/his partners, but also the morale and outlook of field and management personnel. Their impact on patient care, public relations, and the public image of the system can be disastrous.

**Have You Caught Yourself Making Persistently Cynical Remarks?** As with negativity, a cynical attitude is harder to spot in a dispatcher who is normally suspicious and cynical. Even the smallest changes should be carefully noted, both in your own behavior and in that of your colleagues. The cynical person doubts the existence of basic human goodness, and questions the motivation behind every apparently positive action ("What's he after?" or "What does she want?"). This tendency can impact the system in a dramatically negative fashion, since accurate prioritization of call information depends on the call-taker's ability to depersonalize the experience and remain nonjudgmental.

**Are You Frequently Absent or Tardy?** When feelings of dissatisfaction with the job become frequent (due to any or all of the factors described above), certain attendance and tardiness patterns begin to develop. Somewhere in your head, a voice says, "That is not a good place to be. I don't perform well there. It hurts. I don't like it there. I don't want to go there." Some workers try to avoid these bad feelings altogether by missing entire shifts due to real, stress-induced, or imagined illness; others are regularly late for their assigned shifts. Habitual tardiness is a particularly frustrating occurrence for the unenlightened dispatcher, who will find herself/himself unable to get to work on time, no matter what steps she/he takes to try to correct the problem.

**Do You Feel Abused, Unappreciated, or "Picked On"?** When stress levels are dangerously high, the communicator may find routine requests completely unmanageable. A nonthreatening request to correct a minor performance deficit or a simple, minor change in procedure, even when the benefits to the system are immediately obvious, may seem like "the last straw." It is from these employees that the generalized complaints of "They don't pay me enough to do this," and "We do all the work while management just sits around" are most frequently heard. While I'm not completely discounting the possibilities that the employee could in fact be underpaid, and that some members of the management staff could in fact be ineffective, the majority of the time, these comments are cop-outs. "Poor little me" types of complaints are used (whether consciously or unconsciously) because they are broad, general, and very difficult to address and resolve. There is an old story about a man who encounters a problem and complains constantly. When another man passes by and hears the complaint, he quickly sees an easy remedy for the trouble. "Want me to fix that?" he asks. "No, thanks," replies the first gentleman. "I'd rather bitch."

**Do You Catch Yourself Trying to Shift the Blame to Others?** A certain number of mistakes are inevitable in any dispatch center. Many errors may not even qualify as real "mistakes"; they may simply be actions for which suggestions for improvement can be made by the senior dispatcher on duty or by the communications supervisor. At times, however, real mistakes will be made. These will inevitably be identified through the complex and thorough system of checks and balances in place in any responsible communications division. It is a common reaction for the communicator experiencing stress overload to refuse to accept responsibility for her/his actions, and to attempt to shift the "blame" to another employee. This is an understandable and even predictable reaction; if you are already dissatisfied with your own performance, and are blaming yourself for your general feelings of dissatisfaction, then accepting responsibility for one more event may actually be the last straw.

A common variation of this type of stress reaction is the practice of "sandbagging." For example, if someone says to you, "Jane, you didn't give Medic 2 the apartment number on their call," you may reply, "John was conducting personal business on the telephone, and let an emergency phone line ring four times." This response has absolutely nothing to do with the action in question (yours), but is an instinctive and predictable attempt to shift the attention away from your performance and to someone else's.

**Are You Easily Angered?** In times of stress overload and/or burnout, the medical dispatcher may operate with a "short fuse." Reactions of sadness or anger will be seen which are out of proportion to an actual event that took place. This controller will, to the untrained eye, genuinely *appear* to be *"fine"* one minute, only to explode the next. Although personal problems completely unrelated to the work environment are often the factors impacting the dispatcher's stress level, the outcome is the same: The unpredictability of these responses signals a very real stress overload. It should also cause bells to ring and lights to flash in your head, along with a very forbidding voice that repeatedly says, "Warning! Litigation risk! Warning! Litigation risk . . . ."

**Do You Frequently Have Conflicts with Your On-Shift Partners?** As stress levels increase and burnout approaches, the medical dispatcher may experience more frequent problems in getting along with her/his shift partners in the communications center. Partners may voice their belief that a particular controller is not doing her/his share of the work; the affected employee may focus on her/his partners' personal habits or methods of working, and find fault with those habits and methods. It should be noted that when stress overload and burnout begin to affect one medical dispatcher on a particular shift, initially there will be partners who are unaffected; however, those who are unaffected early in the process will not remain so for long.

**Are You Having Financial Problems?** While evidence of

financial difficulty is not necessarily a sign of stress overload, knowledge of financial problems should alert system status controllers to watch for other signs and symptoms, both in themselves and others. When financial problems develop, most of us are not highly successful in dismissing them from our thoughts. This adds to stress we may be experiencing from other sources. The distress spiral can begin, leading to or compounding feelings of dissatisfaction with our jobs. When we need money, the most simplistic solution to the problem is to work more hours. As work hours increase, our fatigue levels increase; concentration lapses cause mistakes, which increase job dissatisfaction and feelings of failure or inadequacy. It is extremely difficult for a person to remove herself/himself from this downward spiral. In this situation, intervention by a supervisor or professional counselor may be indicated.

**Are You Beginning to Narrow Your Perspective?** When no other method of dealing with critically high stress levels is obviously available, many people simply turn off their emotions. At that point where they can no longer deal with several complicated processes at once, they attempt to cope by narrowing their perspectives and concentrating on one subject area or task. Monitor your own behavior and that of your co-workers, watching for these very specific signs:

- *Compartmentalization.* This person very carefully and precisely separates issues concerning work, home life, and so on, and may refuse even to discuss or comment on one area while in one of the other positions. This is an attempt to avoid the confusion and conflict that result when a balance cannot be achieved between different types of demand on time and energy.

- *Depersonalization.* The employee begins to depersonalize to an extreme the events in the workplace. She or he shows a new lack of concern for others: callers, patients, field personnel, ancillary medical staff, and so on. This communicator can no longer afford to make any personal investment at all in the job. The only emotions displayed will reflect consistent negativism, cynicism, sarcasm, anger, and hostility. Attempts at humor are interpreted as insensitive or "sick." The final and most deadly aspect of this phase is seen when no emotion at all is evident. The dispatcher's attitude indicates only apathy.

- *Withdrawal.* This act of "pulling in" or "pulling away" may be physical or emotional in nature. Those presenting the physical side of the process will smile less often. When they do smile, the expression of happiness will only involve changing their facial expressions; it won't come from their eyes. If before, they hugged friends and family or slapped co-workers on the back, they won't do these things any more. When another person inadvertently brushes against them or touches their hands in conversation, the overloaded communicator will pull sharply away. Those who withdraw emotionally will become very quiet; casual conversation becomes an effort instead of a pleasure. The person who previously voiced concern for co-workers and spontaneously offered compliments and encouragement will now be satisfied merely to perform the mechanics of the job without attracting undue attention.

- *Helplessness.* In the final phase of overload and burnout (which occurs literally just before meltdown), the evidence of feelings and behavior patterns described above exist with another element added. The communicator feels hopeless, helpless, and resigned to the situation as it is now. She or he no longer expects circumstances to eventually change for the better. The perception is that any attempt to stop the downward spiral will fail; in the mind of this communicator, there is no light at the end of the tunnel.

Do you reasonably believe that you have identified one or more of the criteria above in yourself or another medical dispatcher in your system? If so, then you have a decision to make. You must decide *not whether to take action, but what action to take.* And you must decide quickly, because these signs and symptoms indicate a person who is in serious trouble. While it's true that an employee displaying any of the behavior just described can be an *incredible* liability to an EMS system, that's not the bottom line. More important than any professional drawback is the fact that the medical communicator in trouble is a valuable human being at risk for serious and possibly permanent emotional damage.

When a problem such as this is identified, the first impulse for most thinking people is to discuss the issue directly with the co-worker. While this is definitely an option, you should be prepared for an unreasonable, hostile, or irrational response. If this person was capable of reacting "normally," you wouldn't be attempting to discuss this difficult subject with her or him. Unless you particularly enjoy pointless, destructive confrontations, it might be wise to refer the matter to a manager with experience in this area, or to a professional counselor.

If you try a face-to-face discussion and make no progress, or if you don't know what to do, you are strongly encouraged to discuss the matter with the communications administrator or other manager *at once.* Recognition of a problem is the first step toward resolving it. It must be an understood element in the relationship between medical communicators and their supervisors that all such discussions will be held in confidence.

It should be the goal of every system's dispatch division to recognize and assist in the management of stress overload for every employee long before the situation reaches a critical level.

## WORDS TO LIVE BY

Occasionally, in times of extreme overload, you may have questions about whether or not you are actually, inherently suited for the profession you have chosen. My guess would be that you are; you simply may not have received the education that you need to make intelligent decisions about your own life and state of mind as they are affected by your job. It is a possibility, however, that a medical dispatcher could make it through the selection and training process, and not have the personality make-up that will allow her/him to continue in the job and remain healthy. *Different personality types are not good or bad, they are simply different.* When you are attempting to gain an overall perspective of your job, your stress reactions, and your degree of satisfaction or dissatisfaction with your situation, first ask yourself these questions:

- Are your expectations of your job and of your own job performance realistic and attainable? Are you throwing more hours at a problem rather than thinking of ways to work smarter? Are you expecting perfection in your own job performance, and "beating yourself up" because you can't deliver it?
- Are you trying to achieve your own personal best, or are you attempting to solve the problems of the world all in one 12-hour shift? If a friend or co-worker shares a problem with you, do you carry it around for days? Do you feel guilty even when a problem and its resolution are completely outside your sphere of influence?

Take a few minutes to be sure that you understand the following simple statements. They may not be exactly what you want to hear during an emotional crisis, but they *are* facts of life:

- You can't help everyone in the world; not today, anyway. There will always be people you can't save.
- Not everything that's wrong can be changed immediately; if you choose to beat your head against this particular wall, all your brains will spill out on the floor, and you won't have any left if you need them later.
- Even when you're performing a noble, honorable task (like medical dispatching), and doing it better than anyone else in the world can, everybody will not love you. Sometimes, your generosity and selflessness will go unnoticed and unappreciated. Never do a right thing or a good thing expecting thanks or recognition; that way, you won't be disappointed. Do it because it's right.

Now follow these simple guidelines:

If it bothers you, change it.
If you can't change it, walk away from it.

## MANAGING STRESS OVERLOAD AND AVOIDING BURNOUT

*"A mind is a terrible thing to waste."*
— *Commercial television advertisement for the United Negro College Fund*

*"Whom the Gods destroy, they first make mad."*
— *Euripides, fragment*

All of the signs and symptoms previously listed that signal impending or actual stress overload and burnout are actually the visible signs of a misguided attempt to cope with unacceptably high stress levels. We naturally, automatically, reflexively attempt to solve our own problems. Without training, many people will choose counterproductive, sometimes destructive techniques to deal with stress overload.

Some of the more common "bad" techniques used to manage stress are substance abuse, using either alcohol or other chemicals; spending an inordinate amount of time watching television; allowing yourself to believe that "there is nothing you can do" (if this is true, then the hopelessness of the situation *saves* you from trying to resolve the problem); releasing stress and expressing frustrations inappropriately, by fighting either verbally or physically with other persons (shift partners, callers, co-workers in other departments, supervisors, family, friends); and/or making constant threats to quit the job. While these solutions are frequently referred to as "bad," they are actually simply uninformed, uneducated attempts to deal with a common problem. With training, you can make more constructive, more informed decisions about how to successfully manage stress and improve the quality of your life.

Positive Stress Management Techniques

Mechanisms to deal with stress quickly become habits. Bad habits are most quickly and easily broken if they are replaced with good ones. Here are some positive techniques with which to replace the negative habits you may have formed:

**Physical Exercise.** Physical exertion is an excellent way to minimize the effects of stress on both your body and your mind. While physical activity gives a definite boost to your physical feelings of well-being, it also improves your state of mind. It is not absolutely necessary that you engage in intense exercise; go for a walk, get some fresh air. It may be that the biggest benefit from this technique is not the actual physical exertion, but simply the change of focus.

**Make Time for Yourself.** By the nature of our jobs, and the nature of our commitments to our jobs, the majority of us do not consistently succeed in our attempts at "leaving the job at the office." We tend to carry our work home with us. Many dispatchers also work on job-related projects at home in their off time. Many are encouraged by family members and friends who are not involved in EMS to tell "war stories." Give yourself days and hours where you engage in activities that are totally non-work-related. Remember the activities that you found pleasurable before you became involved in emergency medicine. Then try doing them again.

**Take Time Off.** If the job is getting to you, take yourself away from it for a while. Even a short vacation usually works wonders in helping you to change and improve your attitude. If money is a problem, look for inexpensive ways to take short trips. The opportunities are out there; you just have to look to find them. Create an adventure for yourself.

**Cut Your Hair, Find a Hobby, Get a Life.** Emergency medical service has a tendency to quickly become an "all-consuming" preoccupation for its participants. It requires a unique dedication and commitment, since both the opportunity and the responsibility to intervene in the case of illness or injury can appear anytime, anywhere. You can't "turn off" your medical training or your superlative abilities to deal with critical situations. You may recall that when you first started in the business, you had any number of friends who were not involved in EMS. If you have been involved in the industry for more than a short period, you may now realize that you spend all your spare time with those whose occupations are related to yours, either directly or indirectly: other dispatchers, EMTs and paramedics, fire fighters, police officers, physicians, nurses. They understand you better than "normal" people do; you have more in common.

*While service in EMS is a good thing, a "right" thing, and a critically, incredibly important thing, it is not the only thing.* Find for yourself friends and activities totally unrelated to emergency medical service. Read. Write. Draw. Paint. Sing. Dance. Take a course in American Sign Language. Have a party for friends from church. Play bingo. Plant flowers in your yard. *Paint your bathroom, learn to scuba, get a real life.*

## ALLOWING FOR CHANGE

*"Things do not change; we change."*
*— Thoreau, "Walden"*

When you resolve to investigate your options and implement changes in your lifestyle to decrease your work-related stress, be careful not to set yourself up to fail. If you map out an extremely structured plan to change and improve your lifestyle, you may set unrealistic goals for yourself. The object of the exercise is to make you feel better, not worse. If you schedule yourself to be at the fitness center every day at 1830 and then don't make it, the end result will be negative, rather than positive. *You will create more stress for yourself.* If you resolve to lose 30 pounds in three months and then get side-tracked and lose only 10, the end result will be feelings of failure, and dissatisfaction with your performance and your life. You should also allow enough flexibility in your plan to accommodate for the possibility of changes in the nature of your own needs. While an evening workout may suit your needs now, those needs or your interests may be different in a month. If you hold yourself rigidly to your original plan (because the new, less stressed, more directed you doesn't want to be a quitter, or because the new, calmer, more tolerant you wants to see the process through to its completion), you are creating more stress than you are relieving. You are setting yourself up to fail. You are setting yourself up to feel bad about yourself.

The problem of stress overload doesn't develop overnight; it cannot be eliminated overnight. In order to change a factor in your life that is making you unhappy, you must first identify that factor. To identify that factor, you must know and understand yourself. That process can take a considerable amount of time. Learn to make small, gradual changes, and then allow yourself enough time to adjust to them. Be patient with yourself. Relax. *There is no one right answer.*

## PROFESSIONAL ASSISTANCE

Enrollment in professional counseling which can be at least partly subsidized by the system is another option made available in many service areas to assist you in dealing with any problems you may be experiencing. Many employee assistance programs offer guidance and help from both professionally trained psychologists and other types of advisors and counselors. While this is still a relatively new resource, I have observed three basic situations in which medical communicators have made use of this option.

The medical dispatcher who has identified in herself/himself some of the warning signs of stress overload may request to be referred to a professional counselor. An employee who already possesses some degree of self-knowledge and some recognition of self-worth may recognize that problems are developing; she/he possesses the conscious desire to avoid or stop the process of the "downward spiral," and utilizes every resource available to resolve problems in an early stage.

The communicator who has exhibited inappropriate behavior that interferes in some fashion with her/his performance of assigned job duties may be mandated into a professional program by the communications administrator. The dispatch administrator or manager ideally serves as the first "sounding board" for the communicator when stress begins to build to an unacceptable level. Whether or not this function is a planned or desired element of the manager's job, in practical reality, this is the way actual situations often develop. When the supervisor believes that the employee's needs have progressed beyond the scope of the department manager's training, education, and ability to provide the employee with the necessary support, the dispatcher may be mandated into a structured program where she/he can receive assistance from those professionally trained, certified, and qualified to provide that assistance. The decision of the administrator to mandate should be made in conjunction with input from other managers as appropriate; however, the particulars of each case and the action taken must remain confidential. This course of action must never be taken lightly, or with "punishment" as the goal. The decision to mandate must be made when the dispatcher's value as a person and as an employee are acknowledged and accepted, and the desires of the manager and the system are to "salvage" a valuable employee, avoid what will be an otherwise inevitably negative end result of a negative process, and continue the communicator's working relationship with the system.

A system status controller who is experiencing general feelings of unhappiness, dissatisfaction, or sadness may access a professional program when she/he is not able to identify the cause. *It should not be required that the cause-and-effect relationship or process be work-related for an employee to utilize the services available from any employee assistance program.* The concern should be for the overall physical, mental, and emotional well-being of the employee, whether or not problem areas are related to the dispatcher's employment. The programs available in many employee assistance programs include individual, family, marital, sexual, financial, and employment counseling. The communications manager should gladly and confidentially assist any dispatcher in accessing the program; however, involvement or notification of the manager should not be a requirement. Any communicator should feel free to contact representatives of the employee assistance program directly.

## CRITICAL INCIDENT STRESS MANAGEMENT

Since it is a relatively new resource, many misconceptions persist about the process of critical incident stress management and intervention. One common mistake is made when system officials assume that only field personnel who were physically present on the scene of a catastrophic event will need professional assistance. Another critical error is made when entire systems recognize the need for debriefing after multiple or mass casualty incidents, but overlook smaller-scale situations which can be just as damaging. I realized early in my involvement in emergency medical service that I could literally wade through blood and guts on trauma calls without experiencing any major emotional discomfort. As long as my patients did not seem to be in much pain and I didn't have to watch the trauma occur, I was fine. One of the worst field experiences I ever had was when I had to stand and watch a psychiatric patient literally hack large pieces of flesh from her own wrists with a pair of dull scissors during a suicide attempt. I have listened while other seasoned field care-givers advised me by radio that they had just witnessed a major motor vehicle accident. The voices of these normally unshakable medical professionals shook uncontrollably as they described the situation and their need for additional resources.

Listening helplessly while a situation goes bad is just as devastating as watching it; in some ways, it may be worse. Some years ago, before I had ever worked in communications, our system held a rape crisis management seminar for pre-hospital care providers. Seminar participants listened to an audio tape provided by a counselor from a local rape crisis counseling center. We listened as a young woman called a police dispatcher for assistance while an intruder broke into her home. She cried and begged the communicator to help her; he had dispatched several units in his system's hottest emergency mode, and then could provide nothing but emotional support while both awaited the patrol units' arrival. The sounds of the forced entry were audible in the background. When the attacker finally reached the caller and she dropped the telephone, we sat with tears running down our faces as we heard the sounds of the actual physical assault taking place. When the tape ended, the counselor asked us how much time we thought we had just spent listening. After several people had guessed 15, 20, and 30 minutes, she told us that the entire tape was only 4 minutes long. It felt like an eternity; it was the single most emotionally devastating thing I had ever heard. Now I do this for a living. What an idiot.

Incidents like the one just described involve only one patient; they do not require multiple unit responses, complicated mass notification procedures, or large-scale mobilization of additional resources. They do not fit the criteria that exist in most people's minds for critical incidents. However, if the potential injury to the medical call-taker is unrecognized and the stress resulting from the event is left untreated, profound and permanent damage can occur.

With experience and education, those calls that will deeply affect medical dispatchers can be identified before they occur. The stress-induced destructive responses of communicators can be predicted, and direct, immediate intervention can be planned for. These are some of the readily identifiable calls after which the communicator may require critical incident debriefing:

- Any situation, like the call just described, where the call-taker bonds quickly with the caller, and actually hears the events causing injury or death taking place;
- Any response to the notification that an employee of the emergency response system has been injured or killed, especially while on duty;
- Any call where complicated or lengthy pre-arrival instructions are given, especially if critical injury, permanent disability, or death results, and most particularly if the patient is a child or if the injury or death was caused by an abusive situation;
- Any situation where the medical call-taker receives emergency notification from or about a friend or family member, particularly when severe illness, critical injury, or death is the result.

In the aftermath of any critical, multiple, or mass casualty incident, stress debriefing may be necessary for the medical dispatchers individually or as a group. As always, open communication between the system status controllers and the dispatch center administrator is crucial. When an incident of this type takes place, the need for assistance can routinely be anticipated, and the signs of impending or actual stress overload observed; otherwise, upon notification that a problem may exist, the dispatch administrator must immediately arrange one or more critical incident stress management sessions for the affected communicators.

## SUMMARY AND REVIEW

1. What are the components of the stress reaction?
2. What is stress?
3. List six stressors unique to the area of medical communications.
4. List eight of the signs and symptoms of stress overload and burnout. Can you identify others not listed in this chapter?
5. What are some of the coping mechanisms people use which are ultimately destructive?
6. List five positive stress management techniques.
7. Does your system offer the availability of professional counseling as part of its employee benefits package? If so, do you know what services are available? If not, do some research; what would the end cost be to the employee and to the system to make professional assistance available?

# Chapter 18

# DISASTER PLANNING

*"Better put a strong fence 'round the top
of the cliff, than an ambulance down in the valley."*
— *Joseph Malines,* A Fence or an Ambulance, *Stanza 7*

*"It is not enough to do good; one must do it the right way."*
— *John, Viscount Morley,* On Compromise

## HOW TO AVOID HOSTING YOUR OWN DISASTER

Although the title of this chapter is a misnomer, I used it deliberately, to make a point. The incidents that we all think of as disasters *don't have to be disasters.* Instead, they can serve as models of efficiency. These events can demonstrate outstanding organizational abilities, flawless interagency cooperation, and the ability to consistently deliver high-quality patient care and rapid transport. The final loss of life can be minimized, and psychological "fallout" for the care-givers, both in the field and in the communications center, can be greatly reduced. The players can emerge from the incident feeling positive, effective, and proud of their cooperative performance.

There are two elements that invariably distinguish professionally managed multiple or mass casualty incidents from full-blown disasters: *thorough pre-planning and controlled communication.*

## WHY WE PLAN BEFORE THE FACT

*Pay attention, please. One more time: In a crisis situation, a planned response is always better than an unplanned response.* The outlook would be dim enough if, without planning, you did the *wrong* thing. However, experience has shown that if you have planned and practiced nothing, the chances are good that when all hell breaks loose, you will be able to do *absolutely nothing.* Take a minute or two to let that picture build in your mind.

*You receive notification of a mass casualty incident. According to the caller, literally hundreds of people are injured and may be dying. You dispatch several units to the incident. Other field crews dispatch themselves. Then, as radio and telephone traffic increases, you become confused. What should you do next? Since you can't decide on a course of action, you sit and wait. You freeze. You can't answer the telephone; someone might need an ambulance, and all of yours are at the MCI. You don't answer radio traffic, because you don't know what to say. Field supervisors are screaming at you over the radio, field crews are asking for scene information and routing instructions, media people are calling for updates, and emergency calls from the rest of your service area are still coming in. The field crews who depend on you to provide them with critically important information have lost their only communications link with the outside world. Again, because you have no idea where to start to sort out this mess, you just sit there, frozen. Eventually, the system administrators get wind of the incident; they arrive to pry your hands from the arms of your chair. When they lift you up, your legs remain flexed at the knees. They carry you outside and prop you up on the curb; then they return to the dispatch area to try and repair the damage you've done. Humiliated, you relocate to an impoverished third-world country to live out your days in anonymous shame.*

*Melodramatic? Sure. Impossible? Don't kid yourself—it's already happened* (well, okay; probably not the part about the third-world country). Communications personnel frequently make either the wrong decision or no decision at all during a multiple or mass casualty incident, quite simply because of inadequate planning and practice.

## THE UNIQUE NEEDS OF MEDICAL COMMUNICATORS

When a large-scale emergency occurs, communications personnel routinely take the most brutal punishment. In most systems, available supervisory and management personnel go to the scene of a major incident; the dispatchers are left to function on their own. They operate in an arena that's like a goldfish bowl.

If a field crew member makes a mistake on the scene, things will sometimes be disorganized enough that no one will notice. If a communicator errs, everyone knows immediately. In addition, tape recordings of the incident will be played and replayed for the entire civilized world as the event is dissected and examined again and again.

Medical dispatchers feel the same sorrow and frustration as field care-givers during a multiple injury event; they frequently feel even more helpless simply because they *are* so completely removed from the scene. While all their years of programming are screaming at them to *"Do something!"* they can't physically do anything to help. Sadly, although the needs of field personnel for critical incident debriefing are now universally recognized, communicators are still often left out of the debriefing process. Left untreated, the psychological and emotional after-effects of a multiple casualty incident can literally result in the termination of the medical dispatcher's career.

## THE HAZARDS OF WORKING IN THE SPOTLIGHT

Any medical professional who aspires to become an accomplished caregiver in the field setting quickly learns one thing: to show off in front of a crowd. Most of us rapidly overcome any initial feelings of shyness and come to enjoy the attention of bystanders. The most confident field personnel develop a real flair for working under intense pressure and close observation. We're doing important stuff, and we want everyone to know it.

In a critical situation, many EMS workers, both in the field and in the dispatch center, unconsciously seek to draw attention to themselves with their radio behavior. The more anxious, out-of-control, and out-of-breath we sound, the more importance others will attach to what we're doing, right? When we're dealing with lots of awful things, then by damn, we want somebody to notice. We are exhibitionists by nature, and we don't believe in suffering silently.

As medical communicators, we've all heard them: those crew members who arrive on the scene of a major incident and proceed to lose their minds. The pitch of their voices wanders, sometimes landing an octave lower than normal, sometimes an octave higher. Their breathing sounds labored, letting us know that they are expending a great deal of physical energy. They forget to turn their sirens off, and shout to be heard. They forget how repeaters and amplifiers work; they believe they have to scream loud enough that we can hear them without the benefits of modern electronics. They speak very quickly, often so fast that no one can understand a word they're saying. They "jump" their microphones, cutting off the first words of their own transmissions. They either babble incoherently (giving us more information than we *ever* wanted to hear), or bark out orders without giving us enough information to make intelligent choices about resource allocation.

Employees who exhibit this behavior are using the only mechanism they know to alert others to the importance of what they're doing. They are reacting to their own mental videotapes. Communicators frequently display this type of stress reaction. As the pace in the dispatch center picks up, they have ways of manipulating their voices to let the field crews know how pressured and overworked they are.

This type of behavior is common and natural; it is also inappropriate and embarrassing, as well as being *completely unprofessional*. It is only displayed by those who have not been educated in the mechanics of the human stress reaction. With practice, emotional *"acting out"* over the radio can be controlled. Armed with the knowledge of when and why it occurs, you can avoid it altogether.

## PLANNING FOR THE COMMUNICATIONS CENTER

These days, a great deal of thought goes into *"emergency preparedness"*. Writing *"disaster plans"* has become a highly defined science. In some areas, degreed professionals are hired from outside industries to write the plans; in others, committees are formed to do the work. Unfortunately, outside professionals sometimes don't understand how the field crews and medical communicators actually do their jobs; and committee members are sometimes selected by title and seniority, not for their relevant experience and education.

Almost every emergency medical service, hospital, fire department, and police department has a disaster plan; many times, the policies and procedures of different agencies *in the same service area* directly conflict with each other. You will find *huge* volumes containing emergency procedures in the offices of agency managers and city, county, and state officials. In many of these extended sagas, you must plod through *several hundred pages* of legal justifications and illustrations of complicated organizational structures before you get to the actual procedures themselves.

Which part of the emergency medical response system is usually notified first of a physical disaster? Which is charged with getting the medical professionals to the place where the sick and injured are? And in which place are you *least* likely to find a concise, usable emergency management plan? You guessed it: in the ambulance communications center.

*If you received a call right now that a major incident with several hundred injuries had occurred in your service area, what would you do? Literally, step by step, what would you do?* In what order would you do the things that had to be done? In a crisis situation, where every decision is time-critical, you don't need to read 200 pages of emergency laws and justifications. You also don't need to be presented with an unlimited series of options. The availability of too many choices can be just as crippling as having no identified options at all. *You need a short list of simply stated tasks, accompanied by current lists of telephone and pager contact numbers and carefully scripted statements for hospital notifications. The middle of a working multiple casualty incident is not a good place to have to make up procedures as you go.*

## THE TEN CRITICAL STEPS

We've recognized all the things you and your system *should not do* to prepare for and function efficiently during a multiple or mass casualty incident. Now let's identify the elements of a successful communications plan for operation during a catastrophic event. The action items that must be accomplished in the communications center can be listed in ten simple steps.

**Step 1: Identifying the Incident.** First, you must equip yourself with the information you need to ensure that your communicators don't overreact or underreact immediately following the initial notification. This means having a thorough understanding of two key phrases.

*A multiple casualty incident can be defined as any event which involves a large enough number of patients (usually more than 5) that the triage, medical care, scene control, and transportation of those patients will significantly stress the emergency response system in its current state.*

Multiple casualty incidents can be situations as routine as motor vehicle accidents with six backboard patients, or as unusual as chlorine gas leaks with thirty victims of inhalation injuries. If the resources available to the system at the time of the incident are not sufficient to efficiently handle the incident, then more resources must be made available. Each system's administrators must identify a specific set of guidelines for its employees to help them make this distinction. The key word in this type of situation is *multiple*.

*A mass casualty incident is usually defined as any situation involving an inordinately large demand for resources to provide triage, medical care, scene control, and transportation of the patient load (usually 200 patients or more).* This is truly "the big one." Some examples of a mass casualty incident include an accident involving a vehicle (passenger train or commercial aircraft) which carries a large number of people, a weather-related event (tornado, hurricane, or earthquake), or an explosion at a large petroleum or chemical processing facility. Please note this word of caution: when you are notified of an incident at any type of business, stop and think, "What time is it?" Ask the caller if anyone is on duty and working in the facility. If the incident occurs at night and a plant utilizes only day shifts, the chance of mass injury is significantly decreased. Remember to ask; in this situation, you can't afford to assume anything. The key word in this type of situation is *mass*.

While these two types of incidents differ in their end results, the same basic procedures should be followed for both. Multiple casualty procedures should usually just be performed on a smaller scale than those required in mass casualty situations. For example, on-duty field operations supervisors should routinely be notified whenever a second unit is required for any scene response. Field personnel on this type of scene may require additional assistance to handle media attention, unruly crowds, equipment recovery, and so on. Administrative or upper management personnel should be notified in the event of third and fourth unit responses for the same reasons on a larger scale. When supervisors and managers are notified, they can provide extra support. Mass casualty incidents require notification and mobilization of all off-duty personnel.

Some incidents are easier to classify than others. In some instances, you will know as soon as you receive the initial telephone call that this will be a mass casualty incident (i.e., "A tornado has touched down in the center of the downtown freeway exchange during rush hour traffic"). In other situations, you won't know the extent of the injuries until your first unit makes the scene. These circumstances require that the on-duty medical communicators weigh the possible patient care and transportation requirements of the incident against the resources currently available to the system. There is no magic number or formula that will automatically tell you when to activate your MCI plan. When in doubt, you should have the option to contact your chief, communications administrator, or chief executive officer for guidance and direction. Again, half the battle is knowing the appropriate questions to ask, asking them, and never assuming anything.

**Step 2. Dispatching the Initial Response.** The second task you must complete is to send help to the incident location. *You cannot permit your emergency notification procedures to delay this initial response.* Dispatch one unit within the same time constraints you would observe for any emergency call. Advise the responding crew of the type of incident and the possibilities for multiple injuries, and request that they provide you with a patient count and scene information as quickly as possible. Send another unit in the direction of the scene in the nonemergency mode to act as a second if needed. Then move a third unit into the area to handle any other unrelated requests for emergency service.

While it seems to be some sort of cosmic law that routine call volume will drop in direct proportion to the number of patients injured in an MCI, I wouldn't bet the farm on it. Get your resources into position to facilitate a rapid mass response and get ready, *just in case.*

It may also be a good idea to temporarily suspend nonemergency patient transports, either while you wait for confirmation of the incident, or while the confirmed incident runs its course.

**Step 3. Designating a Dedicated Radio Channel.** When the incident is confirmed, immediately move all radio traffic relating to the incident to a separate channel. This channel must be a repeated channel, since field crews and supervisors assigned to the MCI must be able to talk to each other.

One communicator should handle all communications occurring on the dedicated frequency. *If you have to call in extra communications personnel to permit this, you should do it now.*

**Step 4. Notifying Your Management or Command Staff.** As soon as an incident involving a large number of patients has been confirmed, the management staff or command structure for your system should be notified. Ideally, the events just described in Steps 1 through 3 will occur in a time frame that will allow you to notify these managers while the first unit is still responding, and before the incident has been confirmed. (In my system, the "Possible MCI" notification means, "Get out of bed and find your jeans." The "Confirmed MCI in progress" notification means, "Get into your jeans, fling yourself into your car, and drive like hell.")

This alert process can be accomplished through a series of telephone calls; however, it will take forever. Not only does each manager have to be called individually, but each has the opportunity to ask questions that you either don't have time to answer or don't yet know the answers to. The utilization of an automated voice mail system or a paging system which allows select groups of persons to be alerted is infinitely more desirable. Whatever method of notification is used, it should be the responsibility of one communicator to keep track of which administrators have acknowledged the notification. If some members of the command structure do not acknowledge receiving the information, additional steps must be taken, as time permits, to contact them.

It's a good idea to prioritize the information in your alert message to your staff, using the same priorities with which you prioritize your ambulance responses. For example, a priority 1 message could indicate a life-threatening emergency; a priority 2 notification could mean an emergency that is not currently life-threatening; and a priority 3 advisory could indicate an information message only, with the call to be returned at the managers' convenience.

Who should be called, and why? What can anyone but the field care-givers and communications personnel do to help in this kind of situation? When a response readiness protocol for managers or commanders has been correctly planned for and implemented, these people can significantly decrease your work load by quickly making additional resources available. *This is how this is supposed to work: managers, administrators, and command personnel should provide support for those people who actually do the work: you, as medical communicators, and your counterparts, those who provide patient care in the field. Managers should make your job easier, not more difficult.*

*The communications manager* should go directly to the dispatch center. Extra hands will be needed to handle increased demands on communications personnel. Phone calls will have to be made and answered. Critical decisions must be made quickly. Even in a system where the dispatch personnel are thoroughly trained and know what to do in every situation, it is comforting and reassuring to them to have their supervisor or manager present.

*The supply and fleet maintenance supervisors* should notify their supply and maintenance techs and proceed to the location where bulk supplies are stored and ambulances not currently in use are parked. Together, employees of these two departments can stock and prepare additional units to be available if needed. Supply technicians can ensure that extra amounts of supplies specifically related to the specific type of incident are placed in the units (portable oxygen delivery equipment for toxic inhalation, bandaging and splinting supplies for explosions, etc.). Fleet maintenance workers can check fluid levels, *including fuel,* for all available units. *Field supervisors* should go directly to the scene of the incident. There, they can assume the responsibilities for triage, leaving field care-givers free to provide patient care. Supervisors can coordinate transportation efforts, ensuring that all members of a single family end up at the same hospital, that no individual receiving facility gets overloaded, and so on. They can deal with jurisdictional disputes, media attention, and the like, thus allowing field personnel to perform the jobs they were trained to do.

*The operations manager and clinical coordinator* should proceed directly to the scene. The actions of field supervisors can be guided by the operations manager; triage, patient care, and transportation efforts can be assisted by the clinical coordinator.

*The public information officer or public relations representative* for the system should go to the dispatch center. There she or he can directly answer inquiries from media reps as they come in. She/he may also elect to pro-actively contact a particular member of the media corps.

*The financial or business manager* can send representatives from her or his office to receiving facilities. There, they can assist field crews with obtaining information for billing and/or documentation. They can help family members by making follow-up calls to determine the whereabouts of specific patients.

*The chief or chief executive officer* may elect to assist efforts on the scene, to proceed to a civil defense command post, or to help make critical decisions from the communications center. The presence of this person in a pivotal area is important not only for the guidance and direction she/he can provide, but also because it increases the chief's or CEO's knowledge of events *as they occur. Nothing is as frustrating to administrators as being publicly "blindsided" by questions about which they have no information, and for which they have no answers.*

Again, system efficiency in this area is greatly improved with pro-active planning and education. Management and command personnel don't have to stand helplessly by during a catastrophic incident; nor are they necessarily doomed to show up on the scene, feel compelled to issue bizarre orders, and make things worse instead of better. The person who regularly fills each supervisory role must know *before the incident occurs* exactly what she/he is to do and where she/he is to go in a crisis situation. If designated roles and areas of responsibility are clearly defined *before the fact,* administrative personnel can actively participate in bringing the incident to its most satisfactory conclusion.

**Step 5. Alerting Area Medical Facilities.** This process should be approached in much the same manner as is the notification of administrative or managerial personnel. If it's possible, a resource count should be initiated even before a major incident is confirmed, for two reasons: first, you will be able to provide information about the capabilities of receiving facilities to your field responders *without delay, as soon as it's needed*; and second, personnel at area medical facilities will have the opportunity to practice their own internal procedures and plan their approach *before the first patients roll through their doors.* This prompt warning of a multiple or mass casualty incident is especially important today, when so many facilities are forced to operate on *divert* or *drive-by* status so much of the time.

As with administrative notification procedures, a "global" or broad-based method of relaying information is needed to efficiently notify medical facilities of a potential or confirmed catastrophic situation. Some EMS systems utilize telephone lines to allow field personnel to speak directly with physicians or nurses in base hospitals. In these systems, an automated voice mail mechanism may be used to simultaneously alert staff members in all base facilities. If your system uses radio channels or a simple radio patch matrix system to relay patient information, you may quickly open a channel to all hospitals simultaneously. *Whatever technology you use, write the script before you have to use it.* This is one situation where you absolutely *must* say exactly what you mean, no more and no less.

If you rely on yourself and your colleagues to make up an advisory statement on the spot, the chances are very good that it won't communicate exactly what you wanted it to. So what happens if you screw up this step? If you do not successfully convey the gravity of the situation, staff members at the receiving facilities may not take the advisory seriously, and may not prepare. If you exaggerate the situation or don't state known particulars clearly enough, hospital personnel may overreact, calling in expensive and unnecessary specialty teams. Virtually every hospital's disaster plan identifies varying degrees of response. Whether your information statement leads hospital personnel to overestimate or underestimate the indicated level of response, the personnel at those facilities will always (and justifiably) see the problem as one caused by an error on your part.

Here's one example of an appropriate advisory statement:

> *"Attention, all base hospitals; attention all base hospitals. Stand by for priority 2 information; stand by for priority 2 information." Allow a 5 10 second delay for hospital personnel to find something to write with and on. "The Acme Ambulance communications center has received notification of a possible mass (note the wording; be very selective about using either "multiple" or "mass," since these two words indicate specific number ranges of patients) patient incident in deep North Middleburg. The report is of a commercial aircraft down. At this time, our first unit is still responding to the scene; the actual existence of the incident is unconfirmed. The number of patients and the nature of the injuries are still unknown."*
>
> *"We are requesting that, as a precautionary measure, you initiate your bed and resource count now. Repeat, we are requesting that you initiate your bed and resource count now. Please do not call the communications center by telephone. Repeat, please do not call the communications center by telephone. A representative of Acme Ambulance will call your emergency department shortly to advise you of the status of the incident and to take down your bed and resource count."*

At this point, it is advisable to repeat the entire message. Remember to speak very calmly, slowly, and clearly. *You can control the stress level of the entire incident, even dramatically impacting the actions and attitudes of hospital personnel, merely by the tone of your voice.* If you impact the attitudes and/or stress levels of the medical teams involved, *you impact patient care.*

When you have repeated the entire statement, you must confirm that each hospital has received and understood it. When utilizing a voice mail system, you may provide a telephone number which hospital personnel may call and leave a voice message. If using a radio channel, you can directly confirm with each facility: "At this time, I will do a quick roll call of base hospitals to make certain that each facility has heard and understood this alert. When I call your facility name, please state your name and indicate that you have received the message. Hospital A, did you receive?" Hospital A will answer, "This is Dr. Smith. Hospital A received and clear." Disconnect Hospital A from the radio channel. Then say, "Hospital B, did you receive?" Hospital B will answer, "This is Dr. Jones. Hospital B received and clear." (Again, understand that hospital personnel can only play by your rules if they know what those rules are. Make sure that they have all the information they need to understand the alert and that they understand what type of information you need before an actual incident occurs.) Continue until all area base hospitals have been cleared. Then say, "Alert message concluded, (give the time). Acme Ambulance Dispatch clear." Your last transmission will establish an audible "time stamp" for the initial alert; this will be very helpful when you review the incident.

If the pace at which the incident escalates is such that there is not time to perform the above procedure before the incident is confirmed, just change the wording to support a confirmed incident. For example:

> *"Attention, all base hospitals; attention, all base hospitals. Stand by for priority 2 information; stand by for priority 2 information." Again, allow a delay for hospital personnel to prepare to copy the information. "We have a confirmed mass casualty incident in deep North Middletown. The initial report was of a commercial aircraft down; we have visual confirmation from our first unit on the scene that a large aircraft is down, and that it is on fire. Our first unit arrived on the scene at 1544. At this time, the number of patients and the exact nature of injuries is unknown, although we can anticipate a substantial number of critical patients suffering from multiple-system trauma, burns, and inhalation injuries. We are requesting that you initiate your bed and resource count now. Repeat, we are requesting that you initiate your bed and resource count now. Please do not call the communications center by telephone. Repeat, please do not call the communications center by telephone. A representative of Acme Ambulance will contact your emergency department shortly to advise you of the status of the incident and to take down your bed and resource count. Please have this information ready in your emergency department." Continue the procedure as outlined above.*

Within 5 minutes of the time the advisory statement is made, one communicator should begin calling back the base hospitals, either by radio or by telephone. *Call the facilities nearest to the incident location first.* In addition to patients transported by ambulance, these hospitals frequently receive "walking wounded," or patients transported by private vehicle. It is in the best interest of good patient care to give these facilities all the assistance you can in preparing to handle their patient load. Next, call the designated trauma and pediatric centers in your area. Finally, contact all remaining facilities capable of receiving patients of emergency status.

When you call the hospitals back, be prepared to:

- Copy down their bed and resource availability
- Provide them with the confirmed nature and location of the incident
- Identify for them the approximate number of patients, and the best available estimate of the number of those who have sustained critical and noncritical injuries
- Identify for them the facilities closest to the incident location
- Identify any special circumstances about the incident which might help the hospitals prepare for the type of injuries they will be called on to treat (chlorine leak = respiratory compromise; explosions = trauma; etc.)

Each facility has its own MCI call-back plan. You should not attempt to direct the call-back efforts of a facility in any way not previously agreed to. Each hospital will decide when to activate its call-back procedures, and to what degree.

**Step 6. Notifying of On-Duty Crews and Adjusting Coverage.** Page or otherwise verbally contact all available units in the system; instruct field personnel to remain in their units and to monitor radio traffic on the main dispatch channel. (Don't be surprised if you can't immediately contact all your available field crews by radio; if you can't raise them on your main dispatch frequency, ask the controller coordinating the MCI traffic to contact them on the channel dedicated to the MCI. They will be listening to this secondary channel, and praying that they're next to be dispatched to the incident.)

Instruct on-duty field personnel to hold all nonemergency radio traffic. Inform them, briefly, of the existence of the working MCI. Route mobile units around areas where other vehicles are responding in the emergency mode. Continue, through coordination with the communicator handling the MCI, to dispatch units to the scene as needed, and adjust unit deployment as necessary.

**Step 7. Identifying and Mobilizing Mutual Aid Resources.** One communicator should call emergency medical, fire, and police agencies near your service area, briefly advise them of the situation, asking them to place their systems on standby, requesting that they move units into your service area for mutual aid, or requesting that they immediately respond their units directly to the incident location. This is an area of communications that, in order to function efficiently during a crisis, requires a great deal of education and preplanning. Sometimes dispatchers and field personnel with other agencies hear only what they want to hear. While you may know that you asked a nearby agency's dispatcher to move her or his available units into your service area to help handle "routine" requests for emergency service unrelated to the MCI, what may actually be happening is that all available units from this neighboring jurisdiction are screaming through your city, past waiting patients, toward the mass casualty location.

If medical helicopter transport services are available in your area, alert their dispatchers to the situation. They may postpone routine nonemergency transports or modify the locations of their available teams to assist you.

If there is a military installation nearby, flight personnel there already have plans in place to facilitate the transportation of large numbers of people. When an incident results in a large number of "walking wounded," military bases can be a valuable resource. City or privately owned buses may also be used to transport large numbers of noncritical patients; this helps keep your ambulances available to provide critical patient care and rapid transportation when needed.

**Step 8. Informing Law Enforcement and Fire Suppression Agencies.** This is another area where you cannot afford to assume anything. Constantly check and recheck to make sure that fire and police departments who should be responding to the incident are, in fact, responding. Their dispatchers should have all the information about conditions on the scene that your communicators have. This is essential not only to ensure effective performance by all responding parties, but to provide for the safety of responding personnel as well.

**Step 9. Assisting Your Field Crews.** While it is never the function of the medical communicator to second-guess crew members on the scene, it may sometimes become necessary for you to assist and temporarily guide field personnel who need your help.

If, as a medical dispatcher, you are also an experienced field care-giver, do you remember your first multiple-patient, multiple-jurisdictional, or multiple-bystander call? *Oh, come on*; everybody who has been the primary care-giver on a field unit for any length of time has had one of these. If you can't remember yours, it's probably because you've blocked the memory out; it is simply too painful to recall.

In Texas (in polite conversation suitable for mixed company), we call these incidents "goat-ropes." If you've ever watched the goat roping competition at a rodeo, you'll immediately see the connection.

A cute little goat is tied to a stake at one end of the arena. A chute explodes open at the other end, and a horse and rider many times the size of the victim descend on the goat with frightening speed. The object of the competition is for the rider to vault off the horse, throw the goat to the ground, and tie the goat's legs together in less time than anyone else. The poor goat tries to escape from this huge thing racing toward it; when it realizes that it can't go anywhere, it just stands there and screams. The most intelligent move I ever saw by the goat was one that didn't wait for the contestant to throw it off its feet. As soon as the chute opened, this little goat screamed bloody murder and threw herself down, sticking all four legs straight into the air. The riders were all laughing so hard, they couldn't have roped her to save their lives; they had to bring in another goat. What can I say? It's a barbaric state.

My first goat-rope in the field was on the scene of a motor vehicle accident. As my partner and I were dispatched, we wondered aloud if the incident location was even within our response boundaries. It was so far south, it took us nearly 15 minutes to get there from our station. We finally arrived to find ambulances from a neighboring community on the scene. There were five or six (it was dark) "walking wounded" immediately visible, and one man lying on the shoulder of the road. I assumed, as did my partner, that the patients and the scene were under the control of medical personnel from the adjacent city; being neighborly people, we pitched in to help them. While my partner strolled off to help round up the patients with minor injuries, I knelt beside the fire fighter who was administering patient care to the man down. I casually asked how I could help him; he gave me a very strange look. Finally, he said, "Well, you could get your cardiac monitor."

"Sure!" I replied. "His must not be working," I told myself as I returned to my unit for the equipment. Only when I arrived back at the patient's side with the monitor did I look around and realize that, first, I was looking at a city limit sign indicating that the call was inside our boundaries; and second, that all the medical personnel on the scene, with the exception of myself and my partner, *were basic life support certified only*. No wonder that poor firefighter had given me such an odd look.

Panicked, I did a quick assessment of the patient. He was pale, cool, and diaphoretic; he quickly became extremely combative. I could neither auscultate nor palpate a blood pressure. Bruising was developing across his chest. His vehicle had struck another car and then a building, head-on; we were many, many miles from the nearest hospital. I called for the medical helicopter to make a scene response.

I placed the patient on high-flow oxygen, put on the anti-shock garment, and popped in two large-bore IV lines. Just as the helicopter landed, my patient regained consciousness, attempted to sit up, and promptly arrested. The helicopter nurse and I knew each other well; she coordinated CPR efforts and moving to the helicopter while I intubated. I yelled through the crowd to my partner to let him know where to come pick me up. Soon we had the patient loaded and took off for the hospital.

The helicopter crews used folding metal backboards. Each backboard had a hook and chain on one side; when we needed to perform CPR in flight, we attached a metal bar with a padded piston on it. By pushing down on the side of the bar closest to us, we did chest compressions. There was only one problem: someone had hooked the bar up to the wrong side of the backboard. With CPR in progress in the cramped interior of the helicopter, I couldn't disconnect the chain and reconnect it properly.

To provide adequate chest compressions, I had to stand up and lean over the patient throughout the flight to the hospital. While we were in flight, the RN reached to hang the IV bags from the ceiling hook. Just then, we hit a little (a little—hah!) turbulence. She dropped both bags of fluid and sat down, hard, in one of the seats. When she did, she landed, hard, on top of the IV bags. The set-up popped off of one of the bags, and I got hit right between the eyes with Ringer's. That stuff really stings when it gets in your eyes. So the helicopter was bumping along, I was still trying to do compressions while my eyes stung and I sobbed, and my friend the RN was sitting in her seat with her hands on her hips and a steady stream of Ringer's Lactate squirting out from between her legs and saying, "Where is that *coming* from?" The helicopter was bumping along, and the pilot was yelling, *"LADIES! SIT DOWN!"* It was just a disaster. It was, politely stated, a goat-rope.

I'm sure you think I digress, but there's a point to all this. I didn't have any idea what the situation was when we arrived on that scene; I didn't want to admit that I didn't know, so I didn't ask. Since I didn't know what I was supposed to be doing, I didn't do anything for quite some time. By the time I finally figured it out and took some action, things were totally out of control—mine or anyone else's. I felt so inadequate as a result of this mess that I have never allowed that situation to happen to me again.

Virtually any EMS response system that has been in existence for any length of time has in place a multiple patient plan for its field care-givers. *How many of them know exactly what that plan is? How many of the personnel responding to the scene of a particular MCI are either new employees, or seasoned field workers who have never been forced to deal with this type of incident before?* New EMTs worry about where to park the ambulance on motor vehicle accidents; they haven't had a chance yet to worry about this type of response. Many, many senior employees with years of experience in the system will never before have been exposed to a mass or multiple casualty incident. And *absolutely nothing*, no amount of study, education, pre-planning, or situational practice, can completely prepare an emergency worker for the emotional impact of an MCI where profound mutilation or multiple deaths have occurred. Although they don't have time to admit it during the incident, these people are going to feel scared, confused, pressured to act, and frequently emotionally overwhelmed. *Your job is to help them.*

Every person who is employed in your system's dispatch center should know what the field MCI plan is, and exactly how it is applied in practice. If the first personnel on the scene don't appear to know what their roles should be, *gently* direct them until they regain control of themselves, until they figure it out, or until field supervisory personnel arrive on the scene to assist them. Using your system's field MCI plan, what is the designated role of the first paramedic on the scene? Who is the designated triage officer? Who should, by definition, be in charge of communications? Anticipate the needs of your first-on crews, and be supportive.

This is a situation in which the communicators have the opportunity to make a *tremendous* impact on the emotional state of field workers. *You don't have to act out and make someone else look like an idiot to make yourself look good.* Don't embarrass those who don't know what to do, or who lose control. Don't bark orders at them, and don't use a perfunctory, sarcastic tone of voice. *Use your voice as a tool to support them and to help them get through this.* Calm, reasonable, and methodical action on the parts of all communications personnel is critical.

Anticipate what the physical needs of the care-givers on the scene may be. Arrange for extra extrication or fire suppression assistance to be available and ready to respond. If the situation suggests that a large number of toxic inhalation or chemical exposure injuries may have occurred, call poison control or your local hazardous materials authorities and ask what physical signs and symptoms field crews may be required to treat. *Then give control back to the field personnel.* Say, "Medic 1, I have additional information available from poison control if you need it." That way, field personnel don't have to admit publicly that they don't have a clue what they're treating. Tell them, "Medic 2, I have additional fire suppression personnel and equipment available from a neighboring service area with an ETA of less than 10 minutes; advise if you need more resources." This changes the perception of the situation from, "They can't handle this by themselves," *to* "Nobody could handle this alone; good judgment dictates that adequate resources be called in to assist."

Anyone who has mastered patient and scene management in the field knows that a patient in crisis suffers first and foremost from the loss of dignity, and the loss of control over her or his own life. Field care-givers in catastrophic situations suffer from these same losses. *Give them back control of the situation; give them back their dignity.* During an incident of this type, every voice transmission you make should subliminally transmit this message to your field crews: "I am here to help. You have a tremendous amount to deal with right now, and you're doing a great job. How can I make that job easier?"

Think about the physical conditions for the crews. Is this incident going to require that some personnel remain on the scene for hours? Is it very hot or very cold on the scene? Should you send relief personnel in to "spell" your first-on crews? Are personnel on the scene thirsty? Can you motivate someone to take food and drink to the site? Do they need their coats, more blankets, more oxygen, more bandaging supplies? *Think of everything you would want someone to do for you if you were on the scene; then just do it.*

**Step 10. Following Up: Critical Incident Debriefing.** If all the elements described above are planned for and incorporated into your response to an MCI, the emotional damage done to the players in your system may very well be minimal. However, it's very important that each individual be allowed the chance to assess her or his own emotional state following the incident. No administrator should ever make the decision that, since the incident went really well, the individuals involved don't require professional assistance. Many times, the only debriefing required can be accomplished in group or round-table discussions among the participants, directed by a professional counselor. Ideally, these discussions should take place within a designated time frame, with the first occurring within 24–48 hours of the conclusion of the incident. Follow-up sessions are recommended days, weeks, or even months later, to allow for the identification and treatment of delayed stress syndrome.

The approach just described is a fairly common, standard method of dealing with the emotional fallout from a critical incident. However, there is more your system can do to be prepared. If you've gotten this far in this text, you are probably an accomplished medical communicator. Those medical dispatchers with experience both in time and in call volume are usually quite adept at identifying increased or negative stress in voices heard over a radio channel. Using this unique talent, you can encourage your system's command or management personnel to implement a planned procedure that will further protect emergency workers from the profound emotional damage that frequently results from participation in a catastrophic incident.

While the incident is taking place, and while your system is still functioning in the crisis mode, you can listen to the voices of your field crews, mid-management staff, and fellow communicators. Sometimes the stress in those voices is subtle and difficult to detect; at other times, the emotional impact of the situation is very obvious. If you have an employee losing control on the scene, that person needs help *right now,* not tomorrow or the next day. Establish guidelines that will indicate to you when you should seek immediate professional help for your system's workers. If your system provides professional assistance for employees as part of a benefits package, that network of helpers can be activated while the incident is still in progress. Work out the details with the counseling group before a major incident occurs; again, each participant in the process must understand and agree to a planned set of procedures. When an MCI does take place, the medical communicators can directly contact your counseling service and request that representatives be sent to receiving hospitals in your service area. Field personnel will have the opportunity to talk about the experience as soon as they arrive at their transport destination. This practice also allows the counselors to identify those employees who should not work the remainder of their scheduled shifts, and those who will be in need of further counseling. Again, as is usually true, the pro-active stance brings the most positive result.

This is one area where you can't give up, and you can't take "no" for an answer. Even if your management or command staff is not progressive enough, or your system not profitable enough to allow for system-funded professional support, there are still avenues open to you. I know of several communities where the debriefing function is accomplished by volunteers. The training and information needed to provide this type of support are always available. Go to the library. Research crisis intervention techniques. Assistance is frequently available from privately funded or government-supported organizations such as crisis telephone "hot lines," rape counseling centers, and family violence shelters. These experts can assist you in structuring a critical incident "strike team," which functions on an on-call basis, and goes where the need is in an emergency. When paid professionals are made aware of the nature of your need, they will often provide training at no cost, and will volunteer their own time.

While this "do-it-yourself" approach is not always optimal, any level of effort is better than none. Sometimes the knowledge that someone cared enough to plan ahead, the realization that others are experiencing similar feelings, and the availability of a compassionate listening ear will go a long way toward lessening the ultimate damage done.

## SETTING PRACTICAL GOALS FOR THE COMMUNICATIONS CENTER

For some reason, the area within and immediately surrounding my system's contractual boundaries seems to experience a large number of these large-scale incidents; in the last few years, we have operated during many, many multiple patient situations, and several mass casualty incidents. Our current communications MCI procedure has been in place about 2 years. Very recently, our medical communicators received the first call for help concerning a fully occupied school bus which had collided at high speed first with an unknown number of other vehicles, and then with a private residence. While the initial information received obviously did not dictate a mass casualty-type response, the potential existed for 20–40 patients; the fact that the majority of those patients could be children increased the probability of hysterical bystanders, media attention, and the emotional risk to all those called on to provide patient care.

I was working in my office when I heard one call-taker receiving and prioritizing the initial notification. As usual, I could hear each word of the conversation as it took place in our dispatch center. When the telephone call was terminated, there were about 5 seconds of hushed discussion among the on-duty controllers; then three heads popped up over three consoles, and three faces looked directly at me. One of them said, "Possible multiple-patient response." The second added, "Loaded school bus into several cars and then a house." The third told me the geographic location of the incident. Then all three communicators, in unison, reached for their console copies of the dispatch center MCI procedural guide. All three heads disappeared, and they went to work.

It was truly a fascinating experience to watch these medical professionals operate. One communicator dispatched the initial response, moved other units into the area for backup, adjusted unit deployment for the entire service area, and continued to handle routine radio traffic on the main dispatch channel. Another took control of the designated channel for the working incident, relayed pertinent information to our responding personnel, and continued to receive and process additional calls about the incident. The third selected up a county fire frequency to monitor the transmissions of a neighboring fire EMS service which was also responding (since the incident occurred on a boundary of our service area), passed on information about conditions on the scene, placed the medical helicopter on standby status, and maintained frequent telephone communications with the dispatcher for the neighboring agency. Working as a team, they notified the system's administrative staff of the situation, advised all base hospitals to initiate their resource count, and called each facility back to complete the hospital poll. *This entire process, including primary and secondary dispatch, the completion of both internal and external advisory statements, functional system adjustment, and the confirmation of available resources, was completed in less than 6 minutes.*

These medical communicators were calm, controlled, and supportive; each kept the others continually informed of what tasks she or he had either begun or completed, and of the information that had been gathered. In less than 6 minutes, they were prepared for virtually the worst possible scenario that could have resulted from this incident. No voice was ever raised. Throughout the incident, no negative stress was ever evident in any dispatcher's voice, facial expression, or body language. It was profoundly obvious that each of these communications experts considered the situation a personal and professional challenge, not a disaster. I answered an occasional nonemergency telephone line; the remainder of the time, I stood with my hands in my pockets, shook my head, and smiled a lot.

## THE ULTIMATE GOALS

These must be the goals of every emergency medical service: to provide the highest possible quality patient care and customer service, and to accomplish that by providing the best possible training, evaluation, and retraining for key personnel (and *all* employees of an emergency medical service are key personnel). How can these purposes be achieved?

At least in part, these goals can be met by recognizing that the communications division must be included in our critical, industry-wide attempt to decrease the loss of life and improve the quality of life; by giving the medical communicators the authority, information, and consequently, the confidence they require to produce exceptional results; and by treating those communicators with the respect and confidence deserved by intelligent, creative, resourceful, and dependable professionals.

## SUMMARY AND REVIEW

1. Look around your communications center. Is there a copy of your service area's disaster contingency plan?
2. If a plan exists for your area, who wrote it?
3. Is it usable for communications personnel?

4. If you received notification of a mass casualty incident in or adjacent to your service area right now, what would you do?

5. What are the ten critical steps in disaster planning for the communications center?

6. Make some telephone calls. Obtain copies of the disaster plans for your city, county, or parish. How much of the information can you use to write your own plan?

7. Maintain current lists of telephone numbers and radio frequencies for mutual aid resources. List the medical capabilities of emergency departments (those equipped with CT scanners, those officially designated as trauma centers, etc.). List office, home, and mobile telephone numbers, along with pager numbers, for your system's management or command staff. Note home and secondary-employment numbers for all field, communications, and support personnel.

8. List the steps your department can take to prepare for a multiple or mass casualty incident. From that list, further refine the action items into short-term and long-term goals.

# GLOSSARY OF TERMS

**Acknowledgment (Total Acknowledgment):** A word or phrase used to let a caller know that what she/he has said has been heard and understood, to encourage the caller to give more information, or to stop the conversation and redirect it.

**ACLS:** Advanced Cardiac Life Support.

**Advanced Life Support:** Pre-hospital care characterized by "advanced" treatment modalities including invasive therapy, drug administration, electrocardiography, etc.

**Attitude:** The mental state, mood, or disposition of an individual.

**Basic Life Support:** Pre-hospital care generally characterized by the administration of "basic" treatment modalities including patient assessment, bandaging, splinting, cardiopulmonary resuscitation, etc.

**CPR:** Cardiopulmonary Resuscitation

**Call Prioritization:** Questioning process that allows the sending of the minimum number of personnel in the safest response mode which will address all the patient's needs.

**Call Screening:** The practice of refusing to dispatch or referring to another agency those calls deemed to be undesirable or noncritical.

**Central Tendency:** The general inclination of a group of test subjects; identification of the central tendency may include the use of mean, median, mode or all three, depending on the area of general knowledge being tested, the test being administered, and how the numbers will be used.

**Clinical Coordinator:** Monitors and works to improve clinical performance by field care-givers. Reviews medical care administered, acts as medical liaison between field care-givers and the other elements of the professional medical community. Supervises activities of the training director and field training officers.

**Comment:** A response by a caller that has no relation to the direct question that was asked.

**Communication:** The act of making contact with the mind of another.

**Communications Supervisor:** Direct-line supervisor for medical communicators. Responsible for attitude, motivation, standard of performance, and direction of communications as a department. Serves as an advocate for the line communicators.

**Concentration:** Close, fixed, or focused attention.

**Confidentiality:** Maintaining and upholding a standard by which something told to one in secret remains a secret, and is kept in confidence.

**Conflict:** Anything that gets in the way of something we want.

**Cooperation:** The act of working together in a joint effort to achieve a common goal.everything from employee dress codes to field care algorithms to billing procedures.

**Customer Satisfaction:** The end product of all efforts in the areas of patient care and customer service.

**Customer Service:** The effort made by any system or company to accommodate the human needs of the customers and clients. Includes everything from employee dress codes to field care algorithms to billing procedures.

**Demand Analysis:** The result of examining and interpreting historical data to determine what past demands on the system have been, and what future demands will be.

**Detrimental Reliance:** Legal concept referring to those situations where one party charges that she/he relied on another party (specifically an EMS system) usually due to a special relationship, to the ultimate detriment of the patient.

**Dispatcher:** One who issues or sends forth; an individual who directs the actions of others.

**Duty:** An obligation; any action necessary in one's occupation or position.

**Emergency Rule:** Generally and traditionally states that a person functioning in an emergency situation cannot be held to the same performance level or the same expectations of conduct as a person who is not functioning in a state of emergency.

**EMS:** Emergency Medical Service.

**Field Operations Supervisor:** Manages and meets day-to-day needs of field care-givers. Interprets, implements, and enforces policies and procedures for field personnel. Provides on-going evaluations of field employees' job performance.

**Financial Director:** Individual or entity responsible for patient billing, collection of accounts, budgeting, data processing, payroll, general data management and recordkeeping.

**First-Party Caller:** The person actually experiencing the problems prompting a call for help; the patient.

**First Responder:** An agency or individual in a position to have reduced response times to emergency incident locations, and trained in a minimum of basic, life-saving medical techniques and procedures.

**Flash:** A sudden, usually unexpected outburst of anger or bad temper.

**Fleet Maintenance Manager:** Responsible for general upkeep of ambulances, maintaining records to satisfy warranty requirements, scheduling preventative maintenance, etc.

**Foreseeabililty:** Legal concept which presupposes that if bad, incorrect, incomplete, or misleading information is given by a caller, the medical communicator will not be held liable for dispatching errors.

**Four Components of Communication:** Reading, writing, speaking, and listening.

**Freak:** The outbreak of hysteria which takes place when a participant or observer on the scene of a medical emergency first perceives that the emergency exists.

**Half-Acknowledgment (Half-Ack):** A word or syllable used to let the caller know that her/his message has been heard and understood. Delivered softly or in a neutral tone of voice, the half-ack allows the conversation to continue in the direction in which it is currently headed.

**High Actual Demand:** The single highest number of calls ever occurring during a reporting period.

**High Average Demand:** The arithmetic mean of a set of numbers, each of which is the highest to occur in a separate and specific four-week time period.

**Hysteria Threshold:** The point at which the interrogator can break through another person's hysteria to control and direct a conversation, allowing the caller to provide the call-taker with useable information and to follow instructions.

**Integrity:** Uprightness, honesty, sincerity.

**Mean:** The average of a set of numbers.

**Median:** The middle number in any distribution, or the point between the two middle numbers.

**Medical Control:** The practice of exercising informed authority over the medical practices and procedures of an emergency medical care provider.

**Mode:** The most common number in any set of numbers. In any set of numbers where no two are identical, the mode will be absent.

**Morale:** The mental condition of an individual or group as their feelings relate to courage, discipline, confidence, etc.

**Motivation:** The inner drive, impulse, attitude, or incentive that leads one to act in a certain way.

**Negligence:** Legal concept that has traditionally only been proven if all four of the following elements are established:
1. That the defendant had a duty to act
2. That duty was breached, either by omission or commission
3. That an injury resulted from the breach of duty, and
4. That there is clear causation.

**Origination:** A word or phrase that identifies a real or imagined critical development on the scene of a call for medical assistance. With the origination, the information flow normally encountered in the call-taking process stops. Until the origination and the event which triggered it have been resolved, no more useful communication can occur.

**PHTLS:** Pre-Hospital Trauma Life Support.

**Patient Care:** The sum of the intervention techniques utilized by medical communicators and the hands-on care provided by field care-givers. Patient care begins the minute that conversation begins with the caller.

**Peak Average Demand:** The arithmetic mean of a set of numbers, each of which is the highest to occur in a separate and specific 10-week time period.

**Peak-load Staffing:** The practice of structuring schedules to provide more available unit hours during times of peak call demand.

**Physicians' Advisory Group:** Panel or board of area physicians, ideally those specializing in emergency medicine. Reviews standing orders, prioritization and pre-arrival protocols, etc., compares these with local, state and national standards, and helps to formulate policies that affect medical care. Reviews selected medical cases and makes suggestions for improvement.

**Physician Medical Director:** Provides overall medical direction. Acts as liaison with other physicians and medical personnel outside the emergency medical system. Issues standing orders for field care-givers.

**Priority Dispatching:** The process by which medical communicators, having received specialized training, use standardized telephone triage interviewing protocols to prioritize requests for medical assistance according to existing needs. The goal is to send the minimum number of personnel in the safest response mode that will satisfy all the needs of the patient and ensure the delivery of the highest quality patient care.

**Production Manager:** Serves as director of unit hour production. Ultimately responsible for all field personnel, maintenance, supply, and scheduling.

**Prudent Action Rule:** Generally states that an individual, acting under a given set of circumstances, must take the same action that any prudent perosn, trained to the same level of expertise and presented with the same set of circumstances, would take.

**Public Relations:** The planned effort to influence public opinion, action, and reaction through examples of good character and demonstration of responsible performance.

**Range:** The mathematical difference between the highest and lowest in any set of numbers.

**Refreak:** The return of hysteria which occurs at predicted points and after specific events during the process of call-taking and remote intervention.

**Remote Intervention:** The process of the administration of specific directions for action given by trained medical communicators to those who call for help.

**Repetitive Persistence:** The practice of repeating a question or phrase over and over in exactly the same tone and at the same volume, in order to break through the caller's hysteria and assist her/him in providing information and following instructions.

**Response Time:** The elapsed time between when a call for help is received and when care-givers arrive on the scene of the incident or the location of the patient.

**Response Time Compliance:** The state in which an EMS response system meets or exceeds the demands of its legal contracts or local standards for maximum response times (a system is referred to as being "in compliance" or "out of compliance" with contract obligations).

**Response Time Exception:** Any response time that exceeds the parameters set for the maximum allowable time for a specific type or priority of call.

**Second-Party Callers:** Persons who are directly involved with the patient.

**Simple Average Demand:** The arithmetic mean of a set of numbers, each of which indicates the number of responses or transports during a specific hour of a specific day during a given length of time.

**Special Relationship:** Legal concept which refers to promises made by one party and beliefs held by a second party, whether or not the first party directly worked to establish or encourage those beliefs.

**Stress:** Strain; pressure; strained exertion. The body's reaction to a basic need.

**Stressor:** Any factor or element that causes a stress-type reaction.

**Supply Supervisor:** Handles inventory control, product testing and evaluation, ordering of both hard equipment and disposable supples. Responsible for routine maintenance of hard equipment.

**System Status Management:** The act of making the most efficent use of whatever resources are available at any given time, and planning effectively so that the resources available will be adequate to meet the demands on the system.

*Glossary of Terms*

**System Status Manager:** Person responsible for maintaining the EMS response system in a healthy state. Identifies, defines, and directs unit hour utilization. Analyzes historical data and predicts future call volume, geographic demand, and staffing needs. Responsible for data management and reporting.

**Telecommunication.** Communication accomplished through the use of an electronic audio and/or visual link.

**Telephone Triage:** The process of asking planned, structured questions of a caller requesting medical assistance, and then analyzing the responses to those questions to determine the needs of the caller and the patient.

**Third-Party Callers:** Persons not in direct contact or in close proximity of the patient.

**Unit Deployment:** The practice of strategically positioning available units as close as possible to the locations where the next calls will come in.

**Unit Hour:** One ambulance, fully equipped, fully staffed, and fully available for any use required by the system, for the time period of one full hour.

**Unit Hour Demand:** Generally, the number of responses or transports accomplished during one specified hour of one specified day over a given period of time.

**Unit Hours Produced:** The number of unit hours scheduled in any 24-hour period, minus those hours lost to maintenance, resupply, personnel issues, etc. The actual number of hours available to the system in a 24-hour period.

**Unit Hours Scheduled:** The number of unit hours scheduled in any 24-hour period.

**Unit Hour Utilization (Productivity):** Measures the percentage of each unit hour during which "work" is being produced (response utilization), or the percentage of each unit hour during which "revenue" is being produced (transport utilization).

**Validation:** In testing, the process of deciding whether or not an individual question or entire examination measures what it was intended to measure.

**Variable Staffing:** The practice of combining shifts of several different types and lengths to provide the number of unit hours needed at any given time.

# INDEX

**Absence, frequent, 210**
Abuse, feelings of, 210
Access, making post selections and, 59
Acknowledgement:
 half-ack, 97
 total, 95–97
Acting out, 223
Action, inconsistency of demands for, 205
Address, obtaining, 109–10
Administrative documentation, 145–46
Adolescents, educating, 157
Advanced life support (ALS), 6
Advancement within department, 42
Advisory statements, 229–30
AIDS, 143
Algorithms:
 clinical treatment, 47
 for telephone triage, 92–93, 164
Alternate controllers, 39
AMA (against medical advice) form, 140
Ambulance placement, strategy of, 57–59.
 *See also* Unit deployment
Ambulance service, 6
Ancillary personnel, roles of, 5–6
Anger, 211
 dealing with caller's, 102–3
Answering telephone, 109
 emergency line, 85–86
 non-emergency line, 86–87
 speed of, 83–84
Applicants, selection of, 165
Assistance, professional, 217–18
Attack and counterattack, 102–3
Attitude(s), 17–24. *See also* Confidentiality
 adjustment of, 100

contributing to customer satisfaction
 through, 158–60
cynical, 210
departmental, 15–16
establishing priorities, 17–18
integrity, 18–19
maintaining positive, 19–24, 86–87
toward media representatives, changing
 one's, 149–51
negative, 209
Attitude surveys, 190–91
Audio recordings, 130, 132, 136–38
 operation of system, 137–38
 optimal structure and use of, 136–37
Audio tape reviews, 186, 198–200
Audits, performance, 163–64
Average, 192
Avoidable errors, 163

**Barriers to behavioral change, common, 154–55**
Behavior modification techniques, 75–77
Belief in one's self, 25
Benefits administrator, 6
Big boss, 1–2
Billings, Josh, 1
Blame shifting, 211
Boredom, 208–9
Brown, Gene, 25
Burgess, Gelett, 44
Burnout, 203, 204, 208–13
 avoiding, 214–16
 signs and symptoms of, 208–13
Bushnell, Nolan, 26

247

Business manager, 228

**CAD system, 114, 119–20, 130–31, 174**
Calculation testing, 187
Call-back plan, MCI, 231
Call demand analyses, using results of, 51, 52–53
Caller(s). *See also* Psychology of dealing with person in crisis
   categorizing, 103
   hostility from, 100, 102–3
   information required from, 86, 109–11
   suggestions to calm, 113–14
Call for assistance, receiving and processing. *See* Receiving and processing call for assistance
Call prioritization, 10, 92
Call received time, 54
Call screening, 10, 92
Call volume, 49, 50
Call volume reports, 145
Canceled runs, 138–39
Candidate:
   assessment standards for, 163
   selection of, 165
   testing of, 174–76
Care-giver, medical communicator as, 124. *See also* Field care-givers
Carroll, Lewis, 9
Casualty incident
   mass, 225
   multiple, 225
Central tendency, 193
Certification:
   CPR, 166
   national, 127
Chain-style unit deployment, 120, 121
Change:
   allowing for, 216–17
   barriers to behavioral, 154–55
Channeling communications, 66
Chart audit/incident investigation requests, 133–34
Chief executive officer, 228
Child personality type, 31–32
Children:
   educating, about EMS, 157
   talking to, 106–7
Choices, system status management and, 47–48
Church groups, educating, 158
"Chute" times, 109
Citizen planning, lack of, 152–54
Civil litigation, time constraints for, 138
Clawson, Jeff, 10, 93, 98
Clinical coordinator, 5, 164, 228
Clinical treatment algorithms, 47
Co-dependent personality, 209
Codes and signals, radio, 116–17
Command staff, notifying of disaster, 226–28
Comment, 97
Commitment to excellence, 146
Communicable diseases, 142, 143
Communication, 73–80. *See also* Radio communications
   basic, 149, 150
   behavior modification techniques for training in, 75–77
   channeling, 66
   difficulty in perfecting, 74–75
   expectations in, 78
   four components of, 73
   spoken word vs. gesture, 79
   telecommunication vs., 77–78
   training vs. natural talent in, 73–74
Communications center, 25–43
   concentration needs in, 13–14
   cooperation in, 40
   critical decisions, making, 42
   departmental standards, setting, 28–30
   disaster planning for, 223–24, 237–38
   location, 27
   overload, 84–85, 125–26
   personality types in, 30–35
   physical layout, designing, 27–28
   protecting dispatcher's position in, 30
   rotating through positions in, 39–40
   scheduling and staffing, 35–39, 50–51
   sense of humor, need for, 40–41
   shift assignments and advancement within department, 42
   steps in designing, 25–26
   types of errors in, 162–63
Communications division, performance standards for, 163
Communications manager, 227
Communications supervisor, 4
Communication testing, 187
Community health, maintaining, 142–45
Compartmentalization, 212
Competitor personality type, 34
Complaints, 87–88, 133, 137
Compliance, response time, 54, 56–57, 69
Computer-assisted dispatch (CAD) systems, 114, 119–20, 130–31, 174
Concentration, levels of, 13–14, 205
Confidentiality, 18–19
   community health concerns and, 142–43
   of medical records, chart audit/incident investigation and, 133–35
   practical guidelines for release of information, 151
   radio codes for, 117
Confinement in work area, 206
Conflict, 102
   attack and counterattack, 102–3
   dynamics of personal interaction during, 21
   with on-shift partners, 211
Console positions, rotating through, 39–40
Consultants, 6
Contact with public, initial, 65–66, 108
Continuing education, 196–98
Controller, system status, 218
Cooperation in communications center, 40
Coordination with other public safety services, 69, 109
Coordinator, clinical, 5, 164, 228
Core shifts, 36
Counseling, professional, 217–18
Counterattack, attack and, 102–3
Co-workers. *See also* Shift partners
   conflicts with, 211
   emotional fallout with, 205–6
CPR certification, 166
Creativity, 25–26
Crews, notifying of disaster, 231

Critical decisions, making, 42
Critical incident debriefing, 219–20, 222, 235–37
Critical incident stress management and intervention, 218–20
Customer satisfaction, 9, 17–18, 158–60
Customer service, 8
Cynical attitude, 210

**Data collection for Systems Status Management, 48–49**
Debriefing, critical-incident, 219–20, 222, 235–37
Decision-making, critical, 42
Dedicated radio channel, designating, 226
Demand:
   high actual call, 50
   high average, 49–50
   peak average, 50
   simple average, 49, 50
Demand maps, 57, 59, 60
Demands for action, inconsistency of, 205
Departmental standards, setting, 28–30
Depersonalization, 212
Deployment, unit. *See* Unit deployment
Deployment plan:
   implementing, 61–63
   writing, 61, 62
Dernecoeur, Kate Boyd, 93
Detrimental reliance, 127
Deviation from protocols, 126–27
Dickinson, Emily, 148
Dictation test, 186–87
Disaster planning, 221–39
   for communications center, 223–24, 237–38
   reasons for, 221–22
   ten critical steps in, 224–37
     alerting area medical facilities, 228–31
     critical incident debriefing, 219–20, 222, 235–37
     designating dedicated radio channel, 226
     dispatching initial response, 226
     field crew assistance, 232–35
     identifying incident, 224–26
     law enforcement and fire suppression agencies, informing, 232
     mutual aid resources, identifying and mobilizing, 231–32
     notifying management or comand staff, 226–28
     notifying on-duty crews and adjusting coverage, 231
   unique needs of medical communicator and, 222
Diseases, communicable, 142, 143
Dispatcher:
   defining, 10
   protecting position of, 30
Dispatch information, eliciting and recording, 109–14
Dispatching response, 119–20, 226
Documentation and reporting techniques, 129–47
   commitment to excellence and, 146
   increased need for, 129–30
   time stamping of status changes and important events, 111, 130–31
   types of, 131–46
     administrative documentation, 145–46
     legal documentation, 135–42
     for maintaining community health, 142–45
     medical information, 132–35
Drop time reports, 145
Dry runs, 138–39
Duty, legal, 124

**Edison, Thomas Alva, 45**
Education:
   continuing, 196–98
   public, 93, 152–58
Effort, levels of, 205
Elapsed call time reports, 145
Elderly, the:
   dealing with elderly caller, 105–6
   educating, 157–58
Elementary school-age children, educating, 157
Eliot, George, 115
Ellington, Duke, 149
Emergency care instructions, providing, 108–9
Emergency medical service (EMS) system:
   ancillary personnel, roles of, 5–6
   commonly used terms in, 8–9
   growth of, 6–7
   historical perspective on, 1, 6
   industry trends, 6–8
   medical communicator in
     new public image, 12–13, 203–4
     roles and responsibilities of, 9–12, 65–71
     special concentration needs in communications center, 13–14
   medical control, importance of, 5
   national performance standards, emergence of, 7–8
   organizational structure, 1–6
     old-style management, 1–3
     progressive, 3–6
   quality assurance (QA) planning, need for, 9
Emergency rule, 125–26
Emergency telephone line, answering, 85–86
Emerson, Ralph Waldo, 18
Emotional fallout from co-workers, 205–6
Emotional involvement, stress from, 207
Emotional overload, rock personality and, 35
Employee involvement, 162
Employees, maintaining confidentiality for, 19
Employee support groups and action teams, 6
EMS vehicles, coordinating movements of, 109
English, radio communication in, 116–17
Environmental control, stress from, 206
Environmental programming, 23
Equipment, knowledge of, 67–68
   testing, 188
Equipment downtime reports, 146
Errors in communications center, 162–63
Escape response to attack, 102
Euripides, 215

Evaluations, performance, 88, 176, 186, 200
Examination, written, 186–89. *See also* Tests, testing
Exercise, physical, 215
Expectations:
   in communication, 78
   of job, 20–22
Experience level, 166
Extended care facility, transporting to, 110

**Fantasies, letting go of one's, 20–22**
Fatigue, perpetual, 208
Feelings, negative, 209–10
Field care-givers, 28–29, 207
   assisting during disaster, 232–35
   concern for safety of, 66
   as dispatchers, 165
   most important personality trait of, 29
   pre-alerting appropriate, 118–19
   providing for, 18
Field operations supervisors, 4
Fighting, 215
Financial concerns, making post selections and, 59
Financial director, 2, 4
Financial manager, 228
Financial problems, 211–12
Fire suppression agencies, informing of disaster, 232
First impressions, importance of, 83–84, 108
First-party callers, 103
Flash, the, 22–23
Fleet maintenance manager, 4
Fleet maintenance supervisors, 227
Following through on call for assistance, 114
Follow-up calls, 85
Foreseeability, 126
Freak occurrence, 99
Fright or flight mechanism, 102
Full-time communicators, 39
Furniture in communications center, 27

**Gabor, Zsa Zsa, 122**
Gallows humor, 204
Geographic considerations in making post selections, 60
Geographic knowledge, 67
   testing, 187
Gesture vs. spoken word, 79
Glossary, 240–45
Goat-ropes, 232–35

**Haircut, 216**
Half-ack, 97
Handicap, working with, 78
Handout material, 198
Hanging up telephone, 88–89
Hazards, physical scene, 143–45
Headsets, teaching, 194
Helicopter transport, medical, 232
Helplessness, feelings of, 213
Hergesheimer, Joseph, 3
High actual call demand, 50
High average demand, 49–50

High school groups, educating, 157
Hiring standards, 28–30
HIV virus, 142
Hobbies, 216
Hold, placing caller on, 85
Hood, Thomas, 65
Hopelessness, 215
Hospital:
   information elicited from, 110
   transporting to, 110
Hostility from caller, 100, 102–3
Hours, work, 36–39, 204–5
Human element, reintroducing, 9
Humor:
   gallows, 204
   need for sense of, 40–41
Hyperventilation, improper identification and management of, 123–24
Hysterical response, components of, 101–2
Hysterical threshold, 92, 98

**Image, public, 203–4**
Incident, identifying the, 224–26
Incident investigation request, 133–35
Independence of field care-giver, 29
Industry trends, 6–8
Inflection in voice, 95–96
Information:
   dispatch, eliciting, and recording, 109–14
   medical, provision of, 108–9
   practical guidelines for release of, 151
   required from caller, 86, 109–11
Initial response, dispatching, 226
Integrity, 18–19
Intelligence testing, 190
Interfacing with other public safety departments, 69, 109
Interim evaluation, 88, 176, 186
Intervention, remote. *See* Remote intervention
Interview, candidate, 167
Interviewing techniques. *See* Telephone triage

**James, William, 47**
John, Viscount Morley, 221

**Key questions, 111–12**
King, Ben F., 209
Knowledge required in medical communicator role, 66–70

**Large-scale emergency.** *See* **Disaster planning**
Law enforcement agencies, informing of disaster, 232
Learning, continuous, 26. *See also* Education
Legal documentation, 135–42
Legal terms and concepts, 124–27
Leopold, Aldo, 154
Lighting in communications center, 28
Listening skills, 74–76
Litigation, 122–24
   danger zones for, 123–24

documentation and, 129–30
legal terms and concepts in, 124–27
physical scene hazards and, 143–45
time constraints for civil, 138
Location, communications center, 27
Locking time clock, 131
Lost and added unit hours reporting, 51–54, 55, 146

**Macho image, 204**
Major media events, 151–52
Malines, Joseph, 221
Management:
  notifying of disaster, 226–28
  old-style, 1–3
  progressive, 3–6
Manual dispatch systems, 131
Maps, demand, 57, 59, 60
Mass casualty incident, 225. *See also* Disaster planning
Mathematics testing, 187
Mean, 192
Measures of variability, 193
Media:
  dealing with, 149–52
  public education through, 156
  stress from attention of, 206–7
Median, 192
Medical cases, key questions for, 112
Medical communicator:
  activities inappropriate to, 71–72
  as care-giver, 124
  nature of, 11–12, 80
  new public image, 12–13
  protecting quality and integrity of position, 30
  roles and responsibilities of, 9–12, 65–71
Medical control, 5, 163–64
Medical director, 5
Medical facilities, alerting to disaster, 228–31
Medical information:
  provision of, 108–9
  reporting, 132–35
Medical Priority Consultants, Inc., 126
Medical testing, 187
Medical training, 165–66
Medico-legal issues, 122–28
  common mistakes, 123–24
  legal terms and concepts, 124–27
  overview of, 122–23
Medicolegal testing, 188
Mental picture of caller's position, building, 103–5
Middle school groups, educating, 157
Military installations, 232
Mode, 193
Morale of field crews, 18
Motivation, 17–24
Multiple casualty incident, 225. *See also* Disaster planning
Mutual aid resources, identifying and mobilizing, 231–32

**National certification, 127**
National performance standards, emergence of, 7–8
Natural talent in communication, 73–74
Negative feelings, 209–10

Negligence, 124–25
Nestroy, Johann, 45
Noise, stress from, 206
Nonemergency call, 110–11
  answering, 86–87
  format for dispatching, 119
  hostility from caller, 100
Nontransport of patient, documentation of, 138–39
No-rides, 138–39
Nursing home, information elicited from, 110
Nursing personnel, 166

**Old-style management, 1–3**
On-duty crews, notifying of disaster, 231
On-line system management, 111
Operations manager, 3, 228
Options, stress from lack of, 207–8
Organizational structure of EMS system, 1–6
  old-style management, 1–3
  progressive, 3–6
Origination, 97
Outrage, Tort of, 125
Overload:
  communications center, 84–85, 125–26
  emotional, 35
  stress, 202, 203, 204, 208–13

**Paging system, 227**
Paine, Thomas, 108
Panic, call-taker's reaction to, 107
Paramedics, 6–7
Parent personality type, 30–31
Parents, educating, 158
Partners. *See* Shift partners
Patient care, 8
  as top priority, 17
Patient management, 235
Patient refusals, 139–40
Patterns, breaking out of one's, 26
Peak average demand, 50
Peak-load staffing, 50–51
Pediatric call, 106–7
"People" skills, evaluating, 26
Performance evaluations, 88
  interim, 88, 176, 186
  routine, 200
  of telephone techniques, 88
Performance standards, 7–8, 163–64
Persistence, repetitive, 98–99
Personal appearance programs, 157
Personality types, 30–35, 209, 214
Personnel, 1–6
Perspectives, narrowing of, 212–13
Physical exercise, 215
Physical layout of communications center, designing, 27–28
Physical scene hazards, litigation considerations and, 143–45
Physicians' advisory group, 5
Physician's office, transporting to, 110
Pick-up time for scheduled transport, 111
Policies:
  communications, 115–16
  responsibility for knowledge of, 66
Positions, rotating through, 39–40
Position statements, 164–65

Positive attitude, 19–24, 86–87
Post move-ups, making, 120
Post selections, making, 59–60
Pre-alerting appropriate field units, 118–19
Pre-arrival instructions, 10
Preparation for training, 197
Preschool age children, educating, 157
*Principles of Emergency Medical Dispatch* (Clawson and Dernecoeur), 93
Priorities, establishing, 17–18
Prioritization, 127, 149
    call, 10, 92
    of information received, 113
    protocols, 112, 113
Priority dispatching, 90, 92–93
Privacy. *See* Confidentiality
Problem calls, 163–64
Procedural instructions, 164–65
Procedures:
    communications, 115–16
    responsibility for knowledge of, 66
Processing call for assistance. *See* receiving and processing call for assistance
Production manager, 4
Productivity, measuring, 63–64
Professional assistance, 217–18
Professional groups, educating, 158
Professionalism, maintaining, 78, 118
Progressive organizational structure, 3–6
Protocols:
    deviation from, 126–27
    litigation and problems with, 123
    prioritization, 112, 113
Prudent action rule, 125
Psychological edge, telephone answering technique and, 86
Psychological testing, 190
Psychology of dealing with person in crisis, 101–7
    attack and counterattack, 102–3
    building mental picture of caller's position, 103–5
    call-taker's reaction to panic and, 107
    categorizing callers, 103
    children, talking to, 106–7
    elderly caller, dealing with, 105–6
    hysterical response, components of, 101–2
Public contact, initial, 65–66, 108
Public education, 93, 152–58
Public image, 12–13, 203–4
Public relations, 148–60
    customer satisfaction, contributing to, 158–60
    dealing with media, 149–52
    defining, 148–49
    public education, 93, 152–58
        common barriers to change in human behavior and, 154–55
        methods of, 156–58
        reasons for, 152–54, 155
        timing of, 155–56
Public relations or public information director, 5–6
Public relations or public information officer, 151–52, 228
Public safety services, coordination with other, 69, 109
Public visibility, stress from, 206–7

Pursuit, 102

**Quality assurance (QA) and quality improvement in EMS, 69–70, 133, 161–201**
    audio tape reviews, 198–200
    candidate selection, 165, 166–74
    continuing education, 196–98
    errors in communications center, 162–63
    group participation and, 200
    importance of, 9
    initial training process, 176–85, 194
    medical control, 5, 163–64
    minimum prerequisite standards, 165–66
    need for, 161
    performance evaluations, 88, 176, 186, 200
    position statements and procedures, 164–65
    remedial retraining, 194–96
    standardization of telephone procedures, 164
    team approach to, 161–62
    testing
        analyzing and interpreting results, 191–93
        candidate, 174–76
        intelligence, 190
        psychological, 190
        written examinations, 186–89
Questions, key, 111–12. *See also* Telephone triage

**Radio channel, dedicated, 226**
Radio communications, 115–21
    acknowledging unit transmissions, 120
    codes and signals vs. plain English, 116–17
    dispatching response, 119–20
    handling routine traffic, 68
    post move-ups, making, 120
    pre-alerting appropriate field units, 118–19
    procedural overview, 117–18
Radio frequency assignments, 117
Range, 193
Range of services, knowledge of, 69
Reagan, Ronald, 95
Receiving and processing call for assistance, 68, 108–14
    answering telephone, 109
    assignment of resources, timely and appropriate, 109
    coordination with other public safety services, 69, 109
    following through, 114
    key questions, 111–12
    nonemergency call, 86–87, 110–11
    prioritization and recording of information, 113
    provision of medical information, 108–9
    suggestions to keep caller calm, 113–14
    third-party limitations, 112
    three essential elements in, 109–10
Recertification, 196
Recordings, audio, 130, 132, 136–38
Refreak, 99–100

# Index

Refusals, patient, 139–40
Reliance, detrimental, 127
Remedial retraining, 194–96
Remote intervention, 68, 163
   defined, 90–91
   failure to provide directions, 123
   legal charges revolving around, 126, 127
Repair of equipment, 67–68
Repetitive persistence, 98–99
Reporting. *See also* Documentation and reporting techniques
   lost and added unit hours, 51–54, 55, 146
   medical information, 132–35
   response time, 54–57, 58
   response time exception, 57, 58
   unusual incident, 140–42
Reprioritization process, 84–85
Requests, chart audit/incident investigation, 133–34
Residence, transporting to, 110
Resource management, 68, 109
   identifying and mobilizing mutual aid resources, 231–32
Respect for elderly caller, 105
Response:
   dispatching, 119–20
   initial, 226
   planned, 221
Response information, legal documentation of, 135–36
Response productivity, 63
Response time, medical importance of, 47, 48
Response time compliance, 54, 56–57, 69
Response time exception, 56
   reporting, 57, 58
Response time reporting, 54–57, 58
Responsibilities of medical communicator, 65–71
Retraining, remedial, 194–96
Reviews, audio tape, 186, 198–200
Rock personality type, 34–35
Rogers, Will, 44
Roles of medical communicator, 9–12, 65–71
Rotating through positions, 39–40
Routine performance evaluations, 200
Run reports, 145

Sadness, 211
Safety, concern for field crew, 66
Sandbagging, 211
Satisfaction, customer, 9, 17–18, 158–60
Scanners, private citizens with, 117
Scene management, 235
Scheduled transports, 110–11
Scheduling, 35–39, 50–51
Scheduling and staffing records, 145
Scorekeeper personality type, 32–33
Screening, call, 10, 92
Second-party callers, 103
Security, 133–35, 137. *See also* Confidentiality
Selden, John, 124
Selection, 166–74
Senior citizens' groups, educating, 157–58
Sense of humor, need for, 40–41
Shakespeare, William, 81

Shift assignments, 42
Shift change miscommunications, 123
Shift partners:
   conflicts with, 211
   cooperation between, 40
   sense of humor in dealing with, 40–41
Shifts, core, 36
Simple average demand, 49, 50
Smile, power of, 23–24
Smith, Alfred E., 123
Solutions, finding second "right," 26
Speaking skills, 74–77
Special relationships, 127
Speed of telephone response, 83–84
Spelling test, 186–87
Spoken word vs. gesture, 79
Staffing, 35–39, 50–51, 145
Standard deviation, 192, 193
Standards:
   departmental, setting, 28–30
   hiring, 28–30
   performance, 7–8, 163–64
Status changes, time stamping of, 111, 130–31
Stout, Jack, 44, 129
Street-corner posting, 60
Stress, 202–20
   common factors in, 204–8
   components of stress reaction, 202–3
   in controller's voice, 118, 119
   defining, 203
   maintaining public image and, 203–4
   management of, 215–20
      allowing for change, 216–17
      from critical incident, 218–20
      professional assistance, 217–18
   personality type and, 214
   signs and symptoms of overload and burnout, 202, 203, 204, 208–13
Stressors, 203, 204
Substance abuse, 215
Suicide, attempted, 104–5
Suitability of post selections, 60
Supervisors, 227
Supply and fleet maintenance supervisors, 5, 227
Surveys, attitude, 190–91
Symptoms, key questions based on, 112
System level, defined, 61
System status, knowledge of, 69
System status controller, 11, 218
System Status Management, 44–64
   call demand analyses, using results of, 51, 52–53
   data collection for, 48–49
   defining, 44
   definitions of common terms in, 49–51
   goals of, 45
   lost and added unit hours reporting, 51–54, 55, 146
   misuse and mismanagement of, 45–46
   productivity, measuring, 63–64
   refinement of, making smart choices in, 47–48
   response time reporting, 54–57, 58
   responsibility for knowledge of, 66–67
   role of medical communicator and, 11–12
   testing of, 187
   unit deployment and post selection, 57–63

System status manager, (SSM), 4

**Talent in communication, natural, 73–74**
Tape reviews, audio, 186, 198–200
Tardiness, frequent, 210
Tattletale personality type, 33–34
Teaching headsets, 194
Teaching techniques, 194
Team approach, 70, 161–62
Technical knowledge, evaluation of, 186–89
Telecommunications, 77
   advanced techniques, 95–100
   communication vs., 77–78
Telephone number of caller, obtaining, 111
Telephones
   mutually accessible, 194
   as tool, 81
Telephone techniques, basic, 81–89. *See also* Receiving and processing call for assistance
   answering emergency line, 85–86
   answering nonemergency line, 86–87
   for communications center overload, 84–85
   forbidden phrases, 81–82
   handling complaints, 87–88
   hanging up, 88–89
   performance evaluations of, 88
   routine traffic, handling, 68
   speed of response, 83–84
   standardization of procedures, 164
Telephone triage, 68, 163
   common objections and misconceptions about, 91–92
   defined, 90
   philosophy of, 91
   standardized algorithms for, 92–93, 164
Television, 215
Temperature in communications center, 27
Tests, testing, 174–76
   analyzing and interpreting results, 191–93
   intelligence, 190
   psychological, 190
   validation of, 191–92
   written examination, 188–89
Third-party callers, 103
Third-party limitations, 112
Thoreau, Henry David, 216
Time clock, locking, 131
Time constraints for civil litigation, 138
Time for oneself, 215–16
Time off, 216
Time stamping, 111, 130–31
Timing of attitude survey, 190–91
Tone of voice, 98–99, 106
Tort of Outrage, 125
Total acknowledgement (ack), 95–97
Training, 127
   communication, 73–77
   initial, 176, 193–94
   medical, 165–66
Training director, 5
Training positions, 166–67
Transport productivity, 63
Transports:
   documentation of no–rides, 138–39
   scheduled, 110–11
Traumatic incidents, key questions for, 112
Triage, telephone. *See* Telephone triage
Trouble-shooting procedures for equipment, 67–68
Typing test, 174

**Unavoidable errors, 162–63**
Unit cancellations, documentation of, 138–39
Unit deployment, 51, 57–63, 120–21
Unit hour, defined, 49
Unit hour demand, 49
Unit Hour Demand Analysis Worksheet, 51, 52
Unit hours reporting, lost and added, 51–54, 55, 146
Unit hour utilization, 63–64
   reports, 145
Unit transmissions, acknowledging, 120
Unusual incident reporting, 140–42
Unusual Incident Reporting form, 140, 141
Unusual incidents as major media event, 151–52

**Vacation, 216**
Validation of tests, 191–92
Variability, measures of, 193
Variable staffing, 51
Variance, 192
Vision, compensating for absence of direct, 78
Voice:
   inflection in, 95–96
   stress in, 118, 119
   tone of, 98–99, 106
Voice-activated recording and playback devices, 136, 137
Voice control training, 23–24
Voice mail, 226–27, 229

**Warner, Charles Dudley, 148**
Wesley, John, 17
Whistler, J. McN., 126
Withdrawal, 212–13
Work area, confinement in, 206
Work hours, 36–39, 204–5
Working in the spotlight, hazards of, 223
Written examination, 186–89
Wundt, Wilhelm, 190

**Young adults, educating, 157**